INCLINED
ELDERS

INCLINED ELDERS

How to rebrand aging
for self and society

RAMONA OLIVER

Cover and interior design: Adina Cucinov, Flamingo Design.
Cover image: Mykhaylo Pelin, 123rf.com
Editing: www.InkDeepEditing.com

TABLE OF CONTENTS

ACKNOWLEDGMENTS

My journey of writing this book has been personally fulfilling. Not only for my own growth, but in large part due to the wonderful new relationships I have developed with over fifty Inclined Elders throughout the United States. They are mentioned individually in the Contributors section at the back of this book and I will treasure them always. Please accept my heartfelt gratitude for so generously sharing your stories; this book could not have been written without you.

I especially want to acknowledge my book consultant and guide, Dr. Liz Alexander, for leading me on this journey. Working with her has been a joyful experience. Liz pushed me ever so artfully and effectively to a higher level for a far better outcome. She always kept me on course. At the outset she indicated we were starting a journey with a supposed destination of Mars but would likely end up on Pluto—and that my flexibility in going where the story needed to take us would make this a stronger book.

I'm also very grateful to graphic artist Adina Cucicov who, through her visual interpretation, brought the concept of

Inclined Elders to life with a stunning cover illustration. My editor, Erica Ellis, was truly amazing at polishing my prose until it shone.

There are so many friends and colleagues who were very supportive with their encouragement and enthusiasm for the book. I thank you and treasure you all.

And finally, I acknowledge the loving support of my family members, all Inclined Elders, who never doubted that I could accomplish this new undertaking, especially Raymond, Suzanne, Chris and Ashley, Steve and Bobbi-Jo, and Ben and Matty.

INTRODUCTION:
WHY EMBRACE AN
ATTITUDE OF INCLINE?

"I could never be content to take my place
by the fireside and simply look on. Life was meant
to be lived and curiosity must be kept alive.
One must never turn his back on life."
~ **Eleanor Roosevelt**

Herb: The Eternal Incliner

Six years ago, when he was ninety-four, Herb and his wife decided to move from their home in Houston, Texas, to an independent living community in Austin so they could be closer to their children. Their first night in the dining room, Herb looked around and exclaimed to his wife, "Oh my God! There's nothing but old people here!" While Herb later told me he'd made that comment in jest, he admitted secretly that he missed the company of friends who are closer to his children's generation.

During our conversation, Herb declared that he has lived a life of continuous Incline and he is still Inclining. Fittingly, his philosophy is in sync with this rhyme I wrote:

I look in the mirror and who do I see,
It's my younger self smiling back at me.
While society dictates a time of decline,
I follow my soul and choose to Incline.

Herb is an exemplar of an Inclined Elder. He is one of the exceptional ones. According to Statista, the average life expectancy in North America for those born in 2019 is seventy-six for males and eighty-one for females.[1] However, many of us are living healthily, physically and mentally, well into our nineties.

For the first time in history we are not only living longer, we also have an important choice to make: commit to a meaningful, purposeful life of Incline as we get older, or believe that a new stage—one of steady decline—is inevitable. This book is a call to action for you to opt for Incline. Not only for your personal fulfillment, but also to help fuel a social "legacy" that increases the number of positive older role models in everyday life. I have written this book to inspire, inform, and challenge you. By the time you reach the last page, I hope you will have made a new choice: to become an inspiring example of a life of Incline so our society relinquishes—once and for all—the notion that aging is synonymous with "decline," "decrepit," "senile," and "over-the-hill."

I want you to choose an attitude of Incline so that, irrespective of how old you are, you continue to climb hills.

WHO ARE INCLINED ELDERS?

We are the women and men who have made a conscious choice to ignore society's negative mindset of "decline" and "over-the-hill" as we age. Instead we embrace a positive mindset of continuing to Incline and climb ever upwards.

While birthdays may be the accelerator for aging, don't let them become the brakes that stop you from continuing to live a full and happy life, as Herb still does at age 100.

Why have Herb, his wife, and I chosen an attitude of Incline? Because we intend to live a life of achievement, meaning, and purpose and not allow mere birthdays to get in the way. And an attitude of Incline will permit us—and you—to do this.

The metaphor of a hill is an apt one to consider as you grapple with the concept of Inclining because hills are surely easier and more enjoyable to climb than steep, lofty mountains. And they still allow for inspiring discoveries and adventures. Some of their pathways may have twists and turns, and there may be the odd bump in the road, but it is important to continue the ascent. Why? Because the vistas on the trek upward are increasingly breathtaking and exhilarating.

Inclined Elders know that there is no need to rush; it's not a race. We take one step at a time so we can pause to smile at the waving wildflowers along the road.

Your attitude determines the potential for your altitude, so a shift in mindset is required, regardless of your age right now. As you awaken to each new day as an Inclined Elder, the sunrise will greet you with a symphony of color applauding your choice to Incline and climb the hill. You will continue to broaden your experience and deepen your joy of life. This is what has happened for me and the people who shared their stories.

Among the fifty plus people ranging in age from 40 to 100 that I spoke to for this book, those with a positive self-perception of aging maintain a more youthful image of themselves. Similarly, the *Journal of the American Medical Association* reported that researchers at University College London posed the question "How old do you feel you are?" to over 6,500 men and women aged fifty-two and above. Seventy percent felt younger than their actual age. Interestingly, eight years later researchers found that 88% of those who said they felt younger than their actual age were the ones who were still alive.[2] Bottom line? Feeling younger may just help you live longer.

Serving as vibrant role models, the Inclined Elders I spoke to for this book are leaving their own unique legacies of wisdom and inspiration for future generations. There needs to be more of us like them to effect real social change. So why not Incline too? There's an amazing view from up here. Come with us and see for yourself.

YOUR TOUR GUIDE

From an early age I've had a curious nature, always receptive to new adventures and learning. After graduating from high school, I travelled throughout Europe and lived in London, England, for a time. Returning home, I began my professional career. I reinvented myself several times by exploring new opportunities, while always seeking challenge and advancement. I soon realized I wanted to apply my inherent desire for continuous personal and professional growth, or Incline, in service to others. Thus, my passion for helping people with their personal growth became a common thread throughout my life: as a human resource manager/director, career coach, and director of outreach for a university, where I promoted lifelong learning and adult undergraduate and graduate programs.

Along the way, I returned to school in my fifties and earned my undergraduate degree. I enjoyed the journey so much I stayed on and earned my master's. My curious and adventurous nature continued into my sixties and my passion for continuous Incline persists. At the age of seventy, I took on the challenge of writing this book. It's now my intention to continue to climb the hill and Incline as I proceed into my eighties, nineties, and beyond, while still exploring as many new adventures as is possible.

Mine is just one way in which a life of Incline can manifest itself because lifelong learning has been such a personal passion. Yet, as you will discover throughout this book, every single person I spoke with has adopted the desire to Incline in their own, unique way.

Over the years, I've worked with hundreds of people to provide them with the tools and support they needed to continue to develop and grow. The gift I've received has always been the glimmer of hope in their eyes as they realized they could overcome their limiting beliefs and self-doubt and attain their chosen goals. It is my intention to serve as your guide as I share the experiences of people just like you. I hope the challenges they encounter, and the strategies, tips, and techniques they use, will inspire you to continue to Incline as *you* age.

WHY THIS BOOK NOW?

From the conversations I've had, several common themes emerged for those living a life of Incline, from which four significant ones surfaced. Incliners:

- Have a positive attitude and mindset about aging
- Live a life of meaning and purpose
- Understand the importance of connections and community
- Realize their legacy is to serve as role models for future generations

The thread weaving these common approaches together was the ability of Incliners to discard their limiting beliefs and summon the courage and confidence to make changes. That's the work. I can provide you with the guideposts to Incline, but you need to be willing to begin the journey and persevere.

The illustrative stories in this book focus on everyday people who are living a life of Incline. Through reading the stories they have shared with you, you will learn about their attitudes about aging and their challenges. You will also discover practical tips, techniques, and strategies for continuing to live a life of Incline. I invite you to develop this legacy gift for yourself. In so doing, you will become more adept at envisioning this new extended life span with meaning, purpose, and new opportunities.

But you are not only going to read about people in their fifties and beyond. In order to capture the attitude of the younger generation towards aging, I spoke with young adults in their twenties and thirties. Research indicates that many of the younger generations have succumbed to society's negative connotation of old age as a period of continuous decline. Many are anxious about facing what they perceive as the doom and gloom of aging. However, those who have had positive older role models in their lives, as demonstrated by the young adults in this book, look forward to continuing their lives as Incliners.

It is my hope you will learn to appreciate how important it is to live with an open mind and not blindly accept society's recommended life path. Thus, the overarching question at the heart of this book is: What does a life of Incline look and feel like and how do you best achieve it?

You may be thinking you've heard all this before: change your attitude, try different behaviors, and buck yourself up—but it never works for you. What is different about this book that you can't get from reading other self-help books about aging? What does this book provide that is not available to you elsewhere?

In *Inclined Elders* I have drawn together experiences from a wide range of men and women aged 40 to 100 to discover what is different about Incliners compared to people who accept—without question or resistance—that life goes downhill as they get older, who believe in the commonly held view in our society that you've just stepped into a new life stage at age sixty or beyond, and things are only going to get worse from here. This is not the message you are going to get from my book. I have taken an approach consistent with Positive Psychology to look at what works in pursuing a life of Incline.

HOW THIS BOOK IS STRUCTURED

Inclined Elders is divided into three sections:

PART 1: ATTITUDE (INTERNAL FOCUS)
What You Need to Change Within You to Lead a More Inclined Life

- Galen will mesmerize you with his "magic illusion" philosophy of life.
- The amazing Miss Lee will share her "recipe for living to ninety-five and beyond."

- Carolyn will tell you how she managed to "dance" even though it was not permitted by her religion and how she continues dancing today at the age of eighty by applying that same principle to other restrictions in her life.
- Kathy will explain how she "laughed fear in the face" and how it helped her to find the courage to live the life she chooses.

I found it fascinating how each of these Incliners put into practice some aspect of Positive Psychology that I had been researching—and they were doing this innately.

PART 2: GROWTH (EXTERNAL FOCUS)
What You Need to Do to Interact Effectively with the External World

- Dorie defines the importance of "relationships" and their positive impact on her life.
- David explains how his philosophy on community and service has shaped his life and allowed him to be a "good man."
- Darlene shares how she refuses to be put into society's "stereotypical box" about aging and how she has benefited as a result.

PART 3: EMPOWERMENT (SOCIETAL FOCUS)
What Society Overall Needs to Do to Create Lasting Change

- Dora shows how she triumphed over her cultural tradition of migrant farm work by earning a bachelor's and then a master's degree, leaving an ongoing legacy of empowerment for her family.
- Polly will share how she overcame her introversion and shyness, chose "self-empowerment," and is now reaping the rewards of serving others by volunteering in her community.

The eighteenth-century English poet William Wordsworth once wrote: "The wiser mind mourns less for what age takes away than what it leaves behind." As you read this book, think about what you would most like to jettison, in order to feel lighter and freer, as you learn how best to live YOUR life of Incline.

PART 1

ATTITUDE

*"The ultimate freedom is
the ability to choose one's attitude
towards certain circumstances."*

~ **Victor Frankl**, author,
Man's Search for Meaning

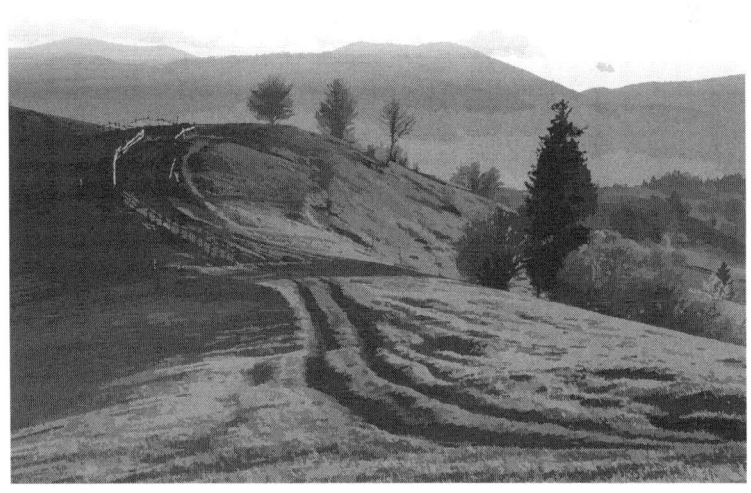

CHAPTER 1

CHOICES MATTER

*"May your choices reflect
your hopes, not your fears."*
~ Nelson Mandela

Poucette: Attitude of Incline

On a cold yet sunny winter day in 1952, a three-year-old little girl set out along a snowy path to explore her new neighborhood. She pushed her favorite doll in her gray buggy, and she had a few crackers tucked into her snow-suit pocket that her mother had given her in case she got hungry. Poucette, nicknamed by her French grandmother for Thumbelina, was wide-eyed and excited about her new adventure. She had just moved with her family to Terrace in northern British Columbia. But unlike her parents and younger brother, who were unpacking and settling into their new home, her curiosity had led her to choose adventure and a desire to explore outdoors.

Sixty-seven years later, that little girl still chooses to look at life with wide-eyed wonder and an attitude of adventure. That is a choice that has never changed for her, regardless of age. Her core essence remains intact. She chooses to live a life of Incline and to continue to climb metaphorical hills. And, yes, that little girl is me. I recently became a septuagenarian, and I'm proud of it.

Whether your inner child is a Tom Thumb or a Thumbelina, or any other adventurous fairy tale character, it's your choice how you live your life. And wouldn't you want it to be as adventurous, relevant, and fun in your sixtieth, seventieth, eightieth, and ninetieth decades as it was in your first? It's possible, as you'll find out when you meet the Incliners and learn how they are meeting the challenges of aging and living life with an attitude of Incline.

I'm sure you've heard countless times, "Just change your attitude." But if it was that easy, we'd already have done it, right? What I'm offering is new and different. I will show you how to examine your current attitude, determine just how much of an Incliner you are, and embrace a series of practical strategies to make that positive shift. For all that and more—read on!

Raymond: Tuning It Out

Clint Eastwood is a cultural icon. He began his acting career in the TV Western series *Rawhide* in 1959, and over the decades he has won acclaim as an actor, producer, director, musician, and political figure, even serving as mayor of Carmel, California, in the 1980s. At the age of eighty-eight, with no sign of retirement in sight, Clint continues to be actively engaged in the work he loves. When asked how he maintains his energy and zest for life at eighty-eight and how others could as well, he responded, "Don't let the old man in."

Which is just another way of declaring that he's living a life of Incline.

Like Clint, my brother Raymond, at sixty-eight, decided not to "let the old man in" and made a choice to live a life of Incline. When asked if there is anything about the external pressures of society's negative mindset that gets him down, he said, "That doesn't affect me at all. If I see some people that are declining, that's their choice. If I don't like what I hear, I tune it out." An avid outdoorsman, he further added, "While I don't climb mountains anymore, I can still enjoy hiking around them. It's simply a matter of modification that I've applied to many life activities."

So, what are some of the different choices and approaches that others have made and how can they help you, too, support a life of continuous Incline? Let's look at the stories of some more of the Incliners.

Galen: Aging as Decline—Reality or Illusion?

Galen recently retired from his position as a technology executive for a healthcare organization and is the author of the book *Unlock the Secrets of Retirement: How to Plan and Achieve a Fulfilling Life in Retirement.* He'd always had a fascination with magic and was curious to see how he might pursue that interest. At seventy, Galen has become quite an adept magician. Performing magic for people young and old has allowed him to bring wonder and delight to others and has injected more joy into his life.

For Galen there is a mystique about retirement being a declining time. His experience is that it's much more positive. He embraces a philosophy of *carpe vitam* or "seize life" rather than simply *carpe diem* or "seize the day." He believes in grabbing hold of retirement and squeezing the most out of it. While our society holds the view that a life of eventual decline is a reality, he says, "It's a reality only if you let it be. I'm a magician. So I would call it the illusion of decline. An illusion, once you know the secret, is not magic. There is a logical, physical explanation. Sometimes it takes a while to discover. Decline in retirement is just such an illusion, but there is a secret to how retirement is really done. You just have to find it."

So, what do we learn from Galen's philosophy? Galen sees our society's negative expectation of eventual decline as an illusion.

I would agree and add further that this is where our ability to make choices comes into play. We all have the free will to determine how we live our lives. I embrace the philosophy of Incline as do the other Incliners from 40 to 100. It's about attitude and the choices we make.

Most magicians strive for "suspended disbelief" when performing magic. Whether it's David Copperfield flying or a lady in a box being sawn in half, the audience knows this isn't happening, but they momentarily suspend that disbelief. Galen takes a different and rather unique approach. He calls it "sell the paradigm" and it's the basis of his performing and creating magic.

Galen has found that the more he reinforces the paradigm in magic, the greater the suspension of disbelief. As he explains, "When we apply this concept to retirement, society is the magician selling the paradigm that retirement is decline." This is reinforced by our society's youth-centric culture, promotion of retirement communities, ageism, and other negative age-related ideas. Is society the magician with a vested interest in selling us an illusion? Unlike the entertainment value provided by the David Copperfields of this world, what happens is detrimental to us, the audience. In this case we are better off eschewing the illusion and creating our own reality.

As a magician, Galen tries to look for the reality. He chooses not to suspend disbelief. And in so doing he has discovered lots of Inclining aspects such as passionately pursuing magic, writing, and speaking. He proactively addresses his health. As Galen asserts, "That is the reality behind the illusion. Reality is not what society is trying to convince us of." So, let's take a lesson from Galen's "paradigm" and choose to shift our thinking to that of Incline and continue to climb the hill.

Speaking of illusions, several notable studies have been conducted that demonstrate how transporting your mind back to a time when you were healthy, happy, and vigorous shifts your physical and mental potential. One, known as the "counterclockwise" study, was conducted in 1979 by Ellen Langer, a Harvard psychologist. Dr. Langer and her team recreated the world of 1959, and the subjects of the study were asked to live as though it were twenty years earlier. A week later, subjects showed improvements in physical strength, mental dexterity, memory, cognition, hearing, and vision. Dr. Langer found that when you believe something will affect you in a specific way, it often will.[1] Her study confirms the power of the mind over the body and demonstrates the multiple benefits of making sure people maintain agency and independence as they age.

Like magic tricks, we can enjoy the reality we create for ourselves a lot more than the reality that society is trying to push at us—"Old is old; get used to it!" In the spirit of "Fake it till you make it," we should eschew this so-called reality—the propaganda, really—of what we are socially conditioned to accept with respect to aging in order to bring the magic of Incline into our lives.

Marie: The Word in Her Heart

Marie, a seventy-seven-year-old former healthcare worker, shared a story in which she reflected on "the word in her heart." As she drove home from a gym workout, a gentleman on a motorcycle honked at her. She realized she had been sidetracked, thinking about her errands for that day, and was driving into oncoming traffic on the wrong side of the road. She immediately turned her vehicle around and into the correct lane. Afterwards she thought: "This has never happened to me. Was this a senior moment or what? I looked back and saw that the man had stopped, and I wondered why he was looking at me. He looked like he was making a call, and so I thought maybe he was calling the police to arrest me. When I arrived home, my reaction was deeply negative, which depressed me for a while. I imagined I was going to have the police come to the door. And then what would happen? So, for a little while, I felt down."

As she often does in situations where she feels a little negative or down, Marie stepped away from thinking negatively, did some gardening, and returned to consider the man-on-the-motorcycle scenario later. She was able to change her way of thinking about that episode in a way that had a more positive slant, which demonstrates her optimistic nature. She changed her thinking and thought perhaps that the man's concern had merely been to make sure she was okay.

In order to shift her thinking, Marie had focused on another activity, gardening. For others, it may be meditation or a walk in nature. A different activity gives your mind the opportunity to refocus so that when you return to the incident, you can reevaluate your thinking.

Marie's story is an excellent one of perspective taking. Of sitting back and saying, "What's another way to look at this that might be different than the automatic reaction." You're ruminating a little bit more and thinking, Okay, there's a different perspective to this. What might that be?

Each facet of Marie's thinking can be explained. According to Dr. Martin Seligman's research, optimists use their personal control and change things with their voluntary actions.[2] Marie's incident had been an isolated event, as she wasn't in the habit of driving the wrong way down a street. She certainly didn't think all people were nasty and judgmental, so she was more inclined to give the man the benefit of the doubt. He was probably just answering an incoming call on his phone, and not calling the police. In addition, she externally personalized the event rather than blaming herself. Seligman proposes that your explanatory style reflects "the word in your heart." It's either a "no" or a "yes"—that is a negative or a positive one—demonstrating pessimism or optimism. This directly relates to an understanding of how your sense of personal control can determine your fate.[3] Additional information about explanatory style is provided in the Resources section at the end of this book.

Martin Seligman is generally considered the father of the modern field of Positive Psychology, the scientific study of what makes life worth living. Happiness and well-being are the desired outcomes. Seligman co-authored *Character Strengths and Virtues*,[4] which is the handbook for this new science. Positive Psychology promotes focusing on the positive aspects of your life—your character strengths—rather than the negative. A link to a tool to identify your strengths is located in the Resources section at the end of this book.

And so, Marie was able to acknowledge the negative emotion yet move through it to a more positive emotion, resulting in an overall positive perspective of the scenario. Marie's "word in her heart" was "yes," and she was able to navigate from an initial negative reaction to a more positive one, thereby resulting in optimism and positivity.

There are those who say that pessimism isn't as "bad" as the negative hype it receives. Granted, there may be some situations where there is merit. I'm not proposing living life as a Pollyanna, the eternal optimist. I advocate that a balance is appropriate (see later discussion on the Positivity Ratio). However, personally, I tend to see more value in living life with a positive attitude.

What is the "word in your heart"? What is your explanatory style? The next time you are confronted with a situation where you are uncertain of your rationale for it, try following this process:

1. Determine the degree to which you feel the negative event will persist—forever or just one incident.
2. Identify whether the event is one that will be ongoing or can be restricted to a specific situation.

3. Assess if you blame yourself or other people or circumstances.[5]

Then see how much better you feel about it.

Lee: Recipe for Living to Ninety-Five and Beyond

At ninety-five, Lee has made a myriad of choices in her life and has created what she refers to as the "Recipe for Living to Ninety-Five and Beyond." Lee is one of the most positive people I have ever met. Her energy and enthusiasm for life are palpable, and it's a joy to be in her company. At a recent lunch to celebrate my upcoming septuagenarian birthday, she gave me some sound advice. She said, "Darlin,' when you tell people you're seventy, I want you to precede your age with J-U-S-T, that is, you're just seventy. And I'm just ninety-five, and we both have many years ahead." Yes, I've now incorporated "just" when I share my age. Thanks, Lee.

On to Lee's recipe.

- **Genes**
  Every doctor who has ever worked on her for surgery, and she's had several, has said she has good genes. But your genes can only carry you so far. While it's a wonderful boost to have good genes, you can destroy the effect of the good genes you've inherited by a lifetime of bad habits.

- **Positive Attitude**
  In sharing this secret, Lee says she is giving you the keys to the kingdom. It's not genes, it's positive attitude.

- **Love**
  Love people. That is the most powerful—it is in every recipe of how to make it into the later ages of life. Love people and be with people. Have a circle of friends and keep in touch often.

- **Lifelong Learning**
  Lee just loves learning. That's key. It's a big one.

- **Sense of Community/Socializing with People**
  Being with people of all ages is also key—both young and old.

- **Spirit**
  The most important thing Lee wants to tell people is that she's been through so much hell, as she calls it, or heartbreak. Altogether in her life she's had a total of thirty years of hell and she's now ninety-five. But what does that tell you? She's had sixty-five years of happiness. That's the way to look at life. The positive. Spirit got her through the unhappy times. She has an anchor in God, but for people who don't believe in a superior being, she recommends calling it hope.

Carolyn: The Dancer

As a young girl, Carolyn grew up with a love of music and a desire to sway and dance to the music in her mind. However, growing up in a strict religious environment, dancing was not permitted. But music within the church was allowed. Carolyn learned to play the organ and because of her growing talent, she soon was asked to play during services. It wasn't until many years later Carolyn realized that as she used the foot pedals, "I was dancing to the music I played." Thus, she chose to follow her heart and express her passion in a unique way not ruled by religious constraints.

Throughout their married life, Carolyn and her husband Max regularly danced together. As she celebrates her eighth decade, Carolyn continues to follow her heart and now dances to the music of her Nia dance classes. (More about Nia and dancing in chapter 3.)

Carolyn is a person who doesn't let life's restrictions stop her from doing what she wants. This is a fundamental aspect of Incliners. No matter what the so-called obstacle or impediment is, Incliners find a way around it. And that is a mindset, an attitude that can be adopted. A choice that can be made. A balance between positive and negative emotions supports Carolyn in living a life of Incline.

Carolyn wanted to dance but felt guilty about it because it went against the rules of the church. However, she didn't feel guilt when she subconsciously "danced" on the organ pedals. Without even realizing it, she had paved another way to get what she wanted and needed. She built resources of innovation that continue to help her. At eighty, Carolyn still "dances on the pedals."

Carolyn's ability to balance the potentially negative events in her life with creative, positive options and attitude is supported by Barbara Fredrickson's work detailed in *Positivity*.

With a positive attitude, Dr. Fredrickson contends you are more open to new possibilities and bounce back from setbacks more easily. As a result of her research, Dr. Fredrickson developed the Positivity Ratio. "It's a way to characterize the amount of your heartfelt positivity relative to the amount of your heart-wrenching negativity." Simply stated, your Positivity Ratio is your frequency of positivity divided by your frequency of negativity or P/N. Fredrickson recommends working towards a Positivity Ratio of 3/1.[6]

Fredrickson likens the Positivity Ratio to a sailboat. The keel beneath the water represents negativity and the sail and the mast above the water represent positivity. While the sail on the mast of positivity catches the wind and provides fuel, it's the keel of negativity that keeps the boat on course. Thus, a balance of both positivity and negativity must be maintained.

I suggest that Carolyn's Positivity Ratio is excellent and floats her boat with an even keel. What is your Positivity Ratio? Take the test. There is a link to the test in the Resources section at the end of this book.

Another aspect of "positivity" is supported by the "Law of Attraction" as detailed by Esther and Jerry Hicks. They contend that the universe is responding to the thoughts you hold, thus you are creating your own reality. The way you feel at any given time is your point of attraction. So, when you choose to feel positive, healthy, vital, and alive, you attract more of all those things into your life.[7] Additional information on the Law of Attraction is available in the Resources section at the end of this book.

Calamitous Cs versus Constructive Cs

What is it about "aging" that is like a self-fulfilling prophesy for so many? I believe there are three conditions that promote negative thinking about aging. They are what I call the three "Calamitous Cs."

Complacency
Complacency for some may conjure up the image presented by Irish poet W.B. Yeats (1865–1939) who, in *When You Are Old,* alludes to being "gray and full of sleep and nodding by the fire." While to others, it may suggest sluggish and lethargic couch potatoes leading sedentary lifestyles who convince themselves they are satisfied with the status quo. Could it be that complacent people settle because of an underlying fear of change? Indeed, complacency can be disguised as contentedness and comfortability. We tell ourselves we aren't making changes because we like things as they are, when really we are afraid to step into the unknown. It is often more about living life on autopilot.

Conventionality
Conventionality is common to those whose sense of safety
is bound up with an adherence to known customs, rules,
and procedures. Yet it also conjures up images of living life
in a way that is absent of any sense of adventure, curiosity,
or creativity. Forever paying lip service to the adage that
"this is the way it's always been done so why change?" Do
we have to accept that aging is all about decline and being
over-the-hill because our society has told us that's just the
way it is? I, for one, and all the Inclined Elders in this book,
disagree wholeheartedly.

Compliance
Compliance may involve buying into the media's and society's propaganda about aging and suggests a conscious yield-
ing to the wishes of others. In other words, acquiescence,
submissiveness, and conformity. I picture a body of people
marching in lockstep in mindless adherence to the dictates
of others and, in doing so, minimizing, if not obliterating,
their own unique individuality. Those who practice compliance are often described as exacting and systematic.

In order to shed the shackles of the "Calamitous Cs" and not
be sucked in by the negative rhetoric of decline in aging,
why not replace them with the three positive "Constructive
Cs": Change, Curiosity, and Courage. Especially if you're
serious about living a life of continuous Incline.

CHANGE

"It's only after you've stepped outside your comfort zone that you begin to change, grow, and transform."

~ **Roy T. Bennett, author,** *The Light in My Heart*

Change can be frightening. It's so safe and secure to be cocooned within the warmth and coziness of a fixed decline mindset. It takes guts to step outside the safety of your comfort zone and peer at the wonderful world that awaits you.

Perhaps you might start making changes in your life with baby steps—literally. As my Pilates teacher advocates, "movement is medicine." Perhaps an early morning walk? A recent study published in the *Frontiers in Human Neuroscience*[8] indicates that routine physical activity can reverse signs of aging in the brain. Interestingly, dancing is the most effective. A very good reason for kicking up your heels! You'll soon find that your steps quickly increase in stride. Keep a diary and daily enter new activities you have tried and accomplished. Celebrate your successes to prove to yourself that change is easier than you think.

Interestingly, the often-held belief that the ability to change is restricted to the young is just not true. Research over the past two decades dispel the myths that the brain cannot grow new brain cells and that older adults can't learn as well as young people. In fact, according to Dr. Gene Cohen, "The brain is more resilient, adaptable, and capable than we long thought."[9] Research has found that:

- The brain continually resculpts itself in response to new experiences and learning.
- New brain cells form throughout life.
- The brain's emotional circuitry becomes more balanced with age.[10]

Further, in his book *The Brain That Changes Itself,* Dr. Norman Doidge discusses the relatively new science of neuroplasticity—*neuro* for the nerve cells in our brains and *plastic* for changeable, malleable, modifiable—and how research has gradually overturned the doctrine of the unchanging brain. He shares numerous case studies that demonstrate how the human brain can indeed change itself.[11]

While it's natural to resist change, with this newfound knowledge, this doesn't have to be your default. Following is just such an example.

Lee: Turning Her Thinking Upside Down

As a young girl Lee dreamed of becoming a fashion designer and entered college with high hopes of accomplishing that goal. While the other students completed assigned art projects quickly, she toiled for hours, sometimes days, to finish her work. Lee began to think that, because it took her so much longer, she didn't have the talent. After graduation, she sadly decided she would never be a designer. She gave up on her dream and instead settled for a job as a secretary for a large oil company where she worked for many years.

And then, at the age of fifty, Lee overheard someone make a comment that turned her thinking upside down. The individual mentioned that Beethoven rewrote his Fifth Symphony thirty-one times before it was completed. In fact, he rewrote all his symphonies many times over. Could that be true? Beethoven! Presumably a genius?

Lee had an awakening in her soul. If it took someone like Beethoven thirty-one rewrites to complete a masterpiece, perhaps talent was more than just a God-given gift. She realized that while talent may come easily to some, perhaps genius level, for others fulfilling a goal may require more work. Lee had incorrectly assumed that if she had talent, she wouldn't have to work so hard. She realized that talent plus hard work equals success. Lee had turned her thinking upside down.

Lee felt she'd been given a second chance to fulfill a dream. She decided to pursue a career as a professional trainer and speaker. She put all her energy into learning how to achieve this goal. Lee recalls: "I had a miserable time getting my brain and mouth to work together. It was hard, but I stuck with it and gradually it all came together. I made the long journey from apprentice to journeyman to master of my craft."

In her sixties, Lee made her mark as an international professional trainer and speaker, motivating and inspiring thousands of people. She later transitioned from speaking and training to coaching and marketing speakers by creating her own bureau, Amazing Speakers and Trainers

International. Lee just celebrated her ninety-fifth birthday surrounded by "amazing" women like herself who continue to live a life of Incline.

The father of American psychology, William James, said, "The greatest discovery of my generation is that human beings can alter their lives by altering their attitudes of mind." By turning her thinking upside down, Lee shifted the inner attitude of her mind to change the outer aspect of her life. Above all, Lee maintains an attitude of gratitude for this valuable life lesson.

Terry: Living in the Now

Terry is a dynamo. A former educator, she formed Women Growing Bolder, and her signature work is now empowering women. At the age of seventy-two she continues to climb metaphorical hills. "The things that can stop me living a life of Incline are either my own inertia, my perfectionism of not knowing how to make a change, or my unwillingness to stop doing the old stuff." Terry nailed three of the top impediments to change. She acknowledged that it's challenging to quit old habits because there is a comfortableness in staying stuck in them. As a workaholic for so many years, she had not developed ways to spend her leisure time—activities just for fun. Realizing this, she is now more actively recreating her future by creating new habits. Like a magician, right? Like Galen, Terry is waving her own magic wand to explore new possibilities and things she has not tried before.

Through the practice of body-centered mindfulness, Terry has learned to keep herself in the present moment, moving forward and not going to the past. She spends time thinking about what is going to make her feel more alive and give her the most joy today. As a planner and a doer, she suggests it's not necessarily knowing what the master plan is but living it out on a more adventurous path. Terry now strives to generate a lifetime of aliveness by living in the now. She identifies new activities that titillate her interests, engage her intellect, and connect her with others.

Mindfulness can be experienced in many ways such as the practice of meditation, yoga, or tai chi. A link to free recordings of guided mindfulness meditations is available in the Resources section at the end of this book.

Another way to experience mindfulness or present-moment awareness is associated with nature. When you find yourself slipping into negative fear-thoughts, go out into nature. This could be as simple as taking a walk, visiting a park, or other outdoor activity. Use the opportunity to focus intently on what is there right now. In a sense, this is a form of walking mindfulness. Focus on the sights, the sounds, the people around you.

The 3-Day Effect,[12] an audiobook by Florence Williams, looks at the science of why being in nature can make us happier, healthier, and more creative. Scientists are finding that the more exposure people have to nature, the more they will benefit from reduced anxiety, enhanced creativity, and overall well-being. *The 3-Day Effect* features cognitive psychologist David Strayer's hypothesis that "being in nature allows the prefrontal cortex, the brain's command center, to dial down and rest, like an overused muscle."[13] The title is a term coined by Strayer, who noticed a significant downward shift in stress levels in group members on a three-day rafting trip. However, research shows even brief interactions with nature can soothe our brains.

Another such practice that is popular in Japan is *shinrin-yoku. Shinrin* means "forest," and *yoku* means "bath." Simply put, *shinrin-yoku* means bathing in the forest atmosphere. Taking in the forest through one's senses. Dr. Qing Li has been studying forest bathing for years and contends that being in nature can ease our stress and worry, restore our mood, and return our energy and vitality. The key to unlocking the power of the forest is in your five senses. [14]

So, let's lace up our walking shoes and get out into nature. I've found that when I walk through a quiet neighborhood park, I focus on experiencing all the sensory opportunities available: a squirrel scurrying across my path, the pungent fragrance of the trees and flora, the sound of birds chirping. Being attuned to the subtle nuances of nature. They all combine to reduce any stress or anxiety I may be experiencing. When I return home, I feel more relaxed, energized, and ready to focus on my projects at hand or the tasks of the day.

I refer you back to my discussion earlier in this chapter about Dr. Langer's study included in her book *Counterclockwise*.[15] Her studies showed dramatic improvements in subjects' health, fitness, and attitude generally through the practice of mindfulness and not succumbing to the mindlessness of an attitude of decline. Thus, subjects of her study were living in the present with an attitude of Incline.

CURIOSITY

"We keep moving forward, opening new doors, and doing new things, because we're curious and curiosity keeps leading us down new paths."
~ **Walt Disney**

Curiosity means waking up each morning with a sense of inquisitiveness, a sense of wonder, and a desire to learn something new. According to George Lowenstein, a professor of economics and psychology at Carnegie Mellon, curiosity is "the feeling that occurs when we experience a gap in knowledge or understanding."[16] That is, between what we know and what we want to know. Like Alice in Wonderland it's good to become "curiouser and curiouser" about the world in which you live and the people that inhabit it. It's a way of making sense of new information that comes into your life.

Curiosity can also help make you smarter because it enhances learning and a youthful sense of fun that can lead to creativity. As Albert Einstein said, "I have no special talents. I am only passionately curious." The key to creativity is curiosity. Being curious enables us to lean into uncertainty with a positive attitude—opening our minds to new ideas. You can expand on your own creativity by developing a love of lifelong learning.

Galen: The Magic of Curiosity

You met Galen, our magician, earlier in this chapter. As an eight-year-old child growing up in a small farming community, magic performances were nonexistent for him. Until one Saturday when a new TV show, *The Magic Land of Allakazam*, appeared. Magic had reached Galen through television! He was in awe! He was hooked! As he thought at the time, "It inspired my curiosity as to how the impossible could be achieved." Galen has been studying and practicing magic ever since.

In his IT career, curiosity provided Galen with the attitude that anything, even challenging assignments, could be done. He just needed to discover how. He approached assignments with the confidence that he would figure it out: sometimes by research, sometimes by asking others, sometimes by creativity. Curiosity also made him more comfortable with change, and there is always change in business and technology. And curiosity helped him to ask questions. How does this change, or this project, fit with the company mission? How can I contribute to making this change successful?

In retirement, curiosity inspired Galen to try new things: going on a cruise, cooking via the "sous vide" method, part-time consulting to help startup companies, producing magic videos, writing a book, and more. Curiosity helps him be open to new experiences.

Galen says, "Magic is part of, and aligned with, my holistic plan for life in retirement: purpose (helping others by creating joy and wonder), hobbies (magic since age eight), exercising my mind (researching and creating new magic effects), networking with others (performing for thousands of people each year), and financial (by generating extra income)." Galen recently won NBC15's Best Magic Trick contest. He regularly performs at local festivals, corporate and private events, summer camps, and retirement communities.

So, from a boy of eight, filled with wonder and curiosity, Galen has evolved to be an "Inclined Elder" magician—lighting up faces of all ages with amazement and joy, and hopefully inspiring that same sense of awe and curiosity in others.

In his book *Unthink: Rediscover Your Creative Genius,* Erik Wahl relates, "In our early years, you and I consistently embodied the key traits that drive constant creativity. Curiosity ruled our senses. Enthusiasm ignited our actions. We did not fear what we did not know—instead we thrived on the process of discovery."[17]

While children are naturally curious, it can serve us in our older years, as well. When we ignite our curiosity and try something new, we are exploring unknown and possibly rewarding territory. As we age, let's continue to challenge our brains and stimulate our thinking. There's nothing to lose and oh so much more to gain. And it's fun!

COURAGE

"Courage is resistance to fear, mastery of fear—
not absence of fear."
~ **Mark Twain**

Embracing change and looking at life with a keener sense of curiosity will lead to living with increased courage. A courage to live life to its fullest.

Courage to live a more meaningful life can be mustered in a myriad of ways. It entails a boldness to take the first step on a new journey and face the fear of the unknown. This recalls Martin Luther King's famous words, "Take the first step in faith. You don't have to see the whole staircase, just take the first step." You can feel fear yet choose to act. A proverb that sums it up is "fear and courage are brothers." Kathy felt fear, yet she chose to laugh in its face and in so doing found the courage to pursue new adventures.

Kathy: Laughing Fear in the Face

Kathy has learned that, as she gets older, she's able to face her anxieties, all those things she's afraid of. Recently, she took a stand-up comedy class. What was her reason for taking the class? "It was to overcome my fear. I just wanted to get over the fear of standing in front of a group of people and feeling like a jerk. It was the hardest thing I've ever done. But I did overcome it." What was Kathy's technique?

She says she just pushed through the fear. But what does that mean?

As a young girl, Kathy was very aware that her maternal grandmother was somewhat fearful. She realized she didn't want to be afraid when she grew up. But once Kathy became a mother, she started noticing her own fears surface. Fearfulness had trickled down, and she had inherited this trait. In fact, there is considerable evidence derived from studies of adopted children and identical twins "that a tendency toward anxiety and fear is a heritable trait."[18]

Kathy would be on the highway in her car and experience panic attacks while driving. She knew she had to get over this. So, when she didn't have her children in the car, she would purposely practice driving on the highways. It worked! Several years later, she became fearful of tunnels and did the same exercise. She drove through tunnels to overcome her fear of enclosed spaces. It worked again! Kathy shared, "It was such a feeling of accomplishment to overcome both of these fears."

Later in life, as a psychiatric nurse for home health, Kathy started having conversations with her patients about her fears and soon learned they also had fears. She expressed, "I realized I was not alone. Discussing my fears with others helped because sometimes when you realize you're not alone, you suffer less. Communicating with others was a win-win for both me and my patients."

Kathy's biggest fear was being vulnerable. Unwittingly, she realized that recognizing one's vulnerabilities is not a weakness. By verbalizing her fears or vulnerabilities, she recognized that our only choice for overcoming fear is engagement. As Brené Brown maintains in *Daring Greatly*, "Our willingness to own and engage with our vulnerability determines the depth of our courage and the clarity of our purpose." You become stronger when you have the courage to embrace your vulnerabilities. You dare more greatly when you acknowledge your fears.[19]

At fifty-six, Kathy continues to "dare greatly" and engage with her vulnerabilities. She has found that in doing so, "I have found the courage to live the life I choose." Kathy is now planning to enroll in an improvisational comedy class.

What vulnerabilities or fears are you blocking that are getting in the way of you living a life of continuous Incline? How can you engage them to find your own courage?

Another option is identifying your character strengths, which is the primary objective of Positive Psychology. A link to a tool to identify your strengths can be found in the Resources section at the end of this book.

Have the courage to follow your heart. In fact, the root of the word courage is "cor," the Latin word for heart. Courage requires us to look into our soul, perhaps be uncomfortable, and make a heart decision.[20] So rather than focus on fear, choose to take action. Make a commitment to do something that inspires you—perhaps piqued by your newfound curiosity and desire for change. Focus on something besides whatever it is that's causing you anxiety and the fear will be neutralized. This cycle will lead to renewed confidence and even greater courage.

Through the application of choices, we need not succumb to the apathy of older age as portrayed by society's negative concept of decline as we age. Rather, we can choose zest and approach life with excitement and energy, not doing things halfway or halfheartedly but living life as an adventure, feeling alive and activated.

As hard as it may seem until you've tried it, it really is your choice whether or not to give in to how late-night comedians, prescription drug advertisements, and the social messages we are bombarded with portray aging. None of which is positive. I have only introduced you to a handful of people, but I promise you there are tens of thousands of similar Incliners out there who are turning their backs on all that nonsense. Bottom line? You'll love life a whole lot more if you join us and continue to Incline.

PERSONAL REFLECTIONS

1. What changes can you make to lead a more Inclined life?
   Consider reviewing the Calamitous Cs and Constructive Cs. Initially take baby steps. Record your progress so you can celebrate each success.

2. What currently piques your curiosity?
   Identify an interest and explore. It could lead to a new area of creativity for you.

3. Identify one of your vulnerabilities. How can you engage with it to embrace your courage and overcome your fear so you can live a life true to yourself?
   Consider completing the Character Strengths and Virtues test in the Resources section at the end of this book to identify your strengths. This is a recommended method of Positive Psychology to overcome your fears.

CHAPTER 2

MAKE EVERY DAY COUNT

*"Gratitude is a powerful catalyst for happiness.
It's the spark that lights a fire of joy in your soul."*

~ **Amy Collette, author,** *The Gratitude Connection*

Betty: The Crystal Bowl

It had been another humid and muggy week in New Orleans, Louisiana, in late August 2005. Betty, a native Louisianan, then sixty-one, and her husband had been tracking the progressive force of Hurricane Katrina. She had lived through and survived Hurricane Betsy. It had hit Florida and the central United States Gulf Coast in September 1965 and brought widespread damage. Was she about to experience another one?

On Sunday morning, August 28, Betty's husband boarded up their home and they hurriedly packed a small suitcase. They left behind clothes, jewelry, pictures, thousands of dollars in US savings bonds, and a beautiful Waterford crystal bowl Betty had recently purchased. She said, "While one may think of materialistic items at a time like this, you just know—get out! There's an imminent threat of the approaching hurricane."

Along with 1.5 million other residents, they fled the city by car. Their destination was Betty's sister-in-law's home on the other side of Lake Pontchartrain and higher ground. A trip that would normally take an hour took four hours. They finally arrived. They were safe.

Katrina slammed into the Gulf of Mexico with winds in excess of 170 miles per hour and on Monday, August 29, it made its way towards Louisiana. Most of the metropolitan area of New Orleans is below sea level. The levee system that held back the waters of Lake Pontchartrain broke under the force of Hurricane Katrina. Eighty percent of the city was underwater.

Several weeks later, when the water had receded, Betty and her husband returned to their home to assess the damage. They waded through the filthy, oil-soaked water. As they neared what was once their dining room, Betty thought of her new Waterford crystal bowl, which she had proudly displayed on her dining room table. Her gaze moved towards the table and she couldn't believe her eyes. The crystal bowl was embedded in the table, weighed down by the flood waters. It was intact and unharmed. It had weathered the storm as she and her husband had. Like the crystal bowl, Betty's spirit was still intact and unscathed by the devastation of the storm and the loss of their home and belongings.

Betty believes that people make their own life—meaning you can worry about so many things but worrying doesn't help. You can't cry over spilled milk. She was so grateful that she and her husband were safe. She was thankful that their house was paid for and they had flood insurance. They could rebuild their life. Betty said, "While I am not a rich person, if you work hard you can obtain the things you need and be very happy. For this I am grateful. I feel I am blessed."

Today, at seventy-four, Betty and her husband have a new home and her crystal bowl is once again proudly displayed on her dining room table. She recently retired from her position as a sales associate at a major department store where she had worked for almost twenty-five years. She continues to be grateful for surviving two hurricanes, as well as many medical issues and operations. Betty is now retired but remains active and lives a meaningful and purposeful life. She greets each morning with a smile and looks forward to enjoying a new day.

Hearing Betty's story reminded me of a quote by Meister Eckhart, a thirteenth century German theologian: "If the only prayer you ever say in your entire life is thank you, that will be enough." I've always loved it because it so simply states the power of gratitude. Being grateful is the most powerful thing you can do to change your life. Gratitude opens the doorway to abundance in your life. How? When you engage gratitude in your life, your ego steps aside. This allows you to connect more deeply with spirit, your true self.

Gratitude is a powerful human emotion. In all forms, it is associated with happiness. By giving and receiving simple thank-yous, we can experience the pleasure and happiness we seek in our lives. It's derived from the Latin word "gratia," meaning grace. When we experience gratitude, we are in a state of grace and thankfulness. Gratitude is a gift that is freely given with no return expectation. It's an attitude you can choose to embrace.

While Betty attributes her sunny disposition to being grateful for a good life and having a positive attitude, there is actual science that identifies how gratitude works and affects the brain. When we express or receive gratitude, our brain releases dopamine and serotonin, two crucial neurotransmitters responsible for our emotions. They make us feel good. They enhance our mood, making us feel happy from the inside out.[1]

Research by leading American investigators of gratitude has shown that gratitude can improve general well-being, increase resilience, strengthen social relationships, and reduce stress and depression. The more grateful people are, the greater their overall well-being and life satisfaction. Grateful people also have a greater capacity for joy and positive emotions. They are happier. The Greater Good

Science Center at UC Berkeley created a gratitude quiz based on a scale developed by psychologists Mitchell Adler and Nancy Fagley.[2] A link to the quiz is provided in the Resources section at the end of this book.

Some simple practices for gifting or experiencing gratitude include:

- Maintaining a personal gratitude journal
- Sending unsolicited notes of appreciation to others
- Scheduling gratitude visits with family or friends to share what you are each grateful for
- Practicing mindfulness
- Taking walks in nature
- Spending time with a "joy buddy"—that special person with whom you share your thoughts of gratitude. Further details on how to develop a "joy buddy" are available in the Resources section at the end of this book.
- Adopting a new practice such as those below that Angela and Carolyn follow

Angela: 3 Good Things

As a successful career consultant, Angela has worked with people on the threshold of career decisions and transition for over two decades. Her business is helping people through change. Her passion is helping people identify their own personal empowerment.

At the age of fifty-four, Angela was going through a major change in her life and was struggling with fear and anxiety. She was building her first home. At first, she had been excited at the prospect of a newly built home. And yet fear and anxiety started creeping into her mind. Instead of feeling anxious, she wanted to feel what she originally thought she would be feeling—joy, happiness, excitement. Fortunately, Angela knew how to make a shift like that, as her work frequently involves helping people who are dealing with anxiety and fear. And she had personally shifted fear this big before. Her tool for shifting fear is a science-based exercise called 3 Good Things developed by Dr. Martin Seligman.[3]

To use the exercise, at the end of each day, you journal three good things that happened during the day and, most importantly, why you consider each a good thing. Dr. Seligman has conducted research that measures happiness in subjects and found that practice of the 3 Good Things exercise can have long-lasting benefits. A further discussion by Dr. Seligman can be viewed online. A link is provided in the Resources section at the end of this book.

And journaling 3 Good Things can have a cumulative effect. The longer you practice, the more benefit you will derive.

Angela's practice of 3 Good Things served her well. She soon was back to feeling joy, happiness, and excitement at the prospect of her new home, which she is now enjoying. And she continues to journal 3 Good Things on a regular basis.

NOTE: A link to Angela's full article is available in the Resources section at the end of this book.

"Rather than use the expression 'I'm blessed' when I express gratitude, I prefer to express that I'm in the blessing." This denotes a deeper sense of gratitude to Angela, almost a form of mindfulness.

Personally, I practice 3 Good Things at the beginning of every day as part of my morning ritual. For me being grateful and expressing gratitude for my previous day's good fortune sets the tone for starting my new day. Try it. Continue it daily. You're sure to reap the benefits.

Carolyn: Blessing and Gift Journal

We met Carolyn "dancing on the pedals" in chapter 1. She believes in paying attention to her physical, spiritual, social, and emotional self. Carolyn stresses that balancing all these areas takes a lifetime of constant perseverance. Sometimes venturing out and trying new things can help with that balance. For example, in her late fifties, she took a journaling class at the Jung Society. The class used Christina Baldwin's *Life's Companion* as a text. There she learned about maintaining a blessing and gift journal.[4] Carolyn started keeping this journal then and she hasn't stopped since.

Carolyn thinks that a blessing and gift journal adds another dimension to a gratitude journal. She includes both blessings she receives and ways she gives back to (and thinks about) others. Carolyn says, "As long as I'm aware that I'm a channel, that I'm being blessed to be a blessing, there is always a constant flow." Now, almost twenty-five years later, at the age of eighty, Carolyn's continued practice of writing down blessings and gifts steers her on a positive course.

Additional information on how to start a blessing and gift journal is available in the Resources section at the end of this book.

I invite you to pause a moment to take stock of all the things you are grateful for. Gratitude may seem simple, but it needs to become a practice if you are to fully reap the benefits. It means not just thinking grateful thoughts periodically. It must become a daily practice. How? Through journaling such as Angela's 3 Good Things or Carolyn's blessing and gift journal. Or the practice of positive affirmations, which is presented in the Resources section at the end of this book. Or reaching out to those in your life you are grateful for and expressing your appreciation and love. Success in your life will be sure to follow. Through the practice of gratitude, you will become more resilient and able to cope with the challenges life may bring.

RESILIENCE

*"Resilience means you experience, you feel,
you fall, you hurt. You fail. But you keep going."*
~ **Yasmin Mogahed, author,** *Love & Happiness*

Betty: The Crystal Bowl—Revisited

Betty epitomizes the definition of resilience, the ability to bounce back. Somewhat like her crystal bowl. She has survived two horrendous hurricanes and several surgeries. And she still retains her positive attitude and outgoing, happy personality.

Recently, Betty required an operation to amputate one of her toes. While recuperating after surgery, she made it her mission to walk the corridors of the hospital, visiting with other patients to brighten their day. One patient was unable to use his hands to eat, and she sat by his bedside and willingly spoon-fed him. The surgery didn't stop her from just "being Betty," that beautiful and caring woman who always puts the needs of others before her own.

So, what is resilience? As defined in Merriam-Webster, resilience is the ability to become strong, healthy, or successful again after something bad happens. To expand, it's that bounce-back attitude—having grit, determination, tenacity. The ability to adapt and respond positively to stress and misfortune. As Seligman asserts in *Authentic Happiness*,[5] the key to building resilience is building your strengths as identified in *Character Strengths and Virtues*.[6] By identifying your character strengths and building on them, you can increase your resilience. To determine your strengths, you can take the survey at the VIA Institute on Character site. A link is provided in the Resources section at the end of this book.

Psychologists have identified some of the factors that make a person resilient, such as a positive attitude, optimism, and the ability to see failure as a form of helpful feedback. Resilience is important because it's critical to our overall well-being. It's connected to our physical, mental and emotional, social, and spiritual well-being.

While there's no magic formula to develop resilience, Dr. Amit Sood, creator of Mayo Clinic's Resilient Mind program and now Executive Director of the Global Center for Resiliency and Well-Being, says there are steps you can take. In his SMART program (Stress Management and Resiliency Training), Dr. Sood recommends incorporating the following five principles into your daily life:

- Gratitude
- Compassion
- Acceptance
- Meaning
- Forgiveness

Cultivating these basic qualities can foster greater resilience and build happiness.[7]

The following story demonstrate the ability to bounce back and continue to live a meaningful and purposeful life after a life-altering occurrence.

Nancy J: Resounding Rebound

At seventy-eight Nancy is still living a full and purposeful life in her third career. She had two successful previous careers, first as a teacher and then as director of a state association. When she retired from her director position, she wanted to become a realtor. She thought it would be a great third career for her as she enjoys working with people.

Yet at the beginning of this new adventure, Nancy was dealt a life-threatening blow. Throughout her life, Nancy always thought she was very healthy because she exercised regularly, ate well, and had close connections with her family and community. So, when she was diagnosed with cancer, she was shocked. Her immediate reaction was that she was grateful for her positive attitude. So she decided to deal with the cancer in the same way. Nancy said, "It was something I had to deal with, and I determined I would be strong and put my positive attitude to work. I held the belief that the ordeal would make me stronger. And I was grateful to have strong support groups—my family, my friends, and my church."

The diagnosis and the ordeal were new learning experiences for Nancy. She realized that when something like cancer comes along it can define your life, if you let it. So much time is required going to the doctor, having tests, having surgeries, doing chemo. Nancy shared, "So, from the very beginning I was very determined to not let it run my life. I continued with my real estate practice, my church work, and other activities."

Nancy faced this life challenge with grace, strength, and resilience and today she has been cancer-free for two years. She continues to live a meaningful and purposeful life and is grateful for her blessings.

Life hits us all with challenges as we age. It's how we choose to deal with them that is important. In *Positivity*, Barbara Fredrickson cites numerous studies where she identified that the most pivotal difference between individuals with and without resilient personality styles is their degree of positivity. "It was the secret of their success. It was the mechanism behind their lesser depression and their greater psychological growth. In short, resilience and positivity go hand in hand. Without positivity, there is no rebound."[8]

Nancy embraces positivity in all aspects of her life and thus demonstrates resilience in facing life's challenges. She displays the two most powerful attributes of resilient people: gratitude and a feeling of control. Renowned expert, Dr. Robert Brooks, has conducted many studies on resilience. He has found that people who are resilient believe they have control over their lives. Rather than having a victim mentality, they focus on what they can do. In numerous studies he has also found that the most discernible difference between individuals who show resilience and those who do not is that the resilient group practiced more gratitude.[9] I'd say that's a great reason to incorporate more gratitude in your daily life.

PURPOSE

"The heart of human excellence often begins to beat when you discover a pursuit that absorbs you, frees you, challenges you, or gives you a sense of meaning, joy, or passion."
~ **Terry Orlick, founder,** Zone of Excellence

BJ: Allow, Accept, Embrace

When I think of BJ, I think of the word serene. Why? Because she is so at peace with herself. She is calm, untroubled, tranquil. She is comfortable in her own skin. BJ derives great joy from sharing her knowledge and herself with others. I am so grateful that she shared the story of the path to her purpose with me.

As a young girl, BJ witnessed her mother's decline and self-destruction. Once a very beautiful woman, excessive drinking, smoking, and eventually a debilitating medical condition caused her deterioration in her thirties. BJ saw the pain and suffering it caused to those around her. Her mother died at sixty-four. BJ shared, "On her deathbed she told me not to wait until the last twenty minutes of my life to realize what life is about and what my purpose is."

That was a pivotal moment for BJ: "It began an internal dialogue to identify my path of spiritual enlightenment—a desire to delve more deeply into understanding my purpose." Many years later, BJ is now an international best-selling author and inspirational teacher with over thirty years' experience in spiritual and psychological instruction. She works with individuals, families, communities, schools, and delinquent youth. She serves as a guide to support people as they embark on their own personal voyage.

Now, at sixty-eight, BJ is an ambassador of the Gene Keys: Unlocking the Higher Purpose Hidden in Your DNA system pioneered by Richard Rudd. She is an expert of the Gene Keys and Enneagram teaching programs. BJ gives freely of her time to help others to explore themselves and identify their life purpose.

One of the tools she attributes most for her successful journey is the 3 Phases of Transformation contained in the teachings of the Gene Keys.[10] They are:

- **Phase 1—Allowing**
  Allowing is when you become aware that something is troubling you. Initially, you don't have to like it or accept it. Just allow it. Allowing is generous. You simply keep seeing it regardless of how uncomfortable it makes you feel.

- **Phase 2—Accepting**
  Accepting is deeper than allowing. After some time, allowing transforms to accepting. Accepting is powerful. It means your awareness can catch you in the act.

- **Phase 3—Embracing**
  Embracing is complete transformation. When you have embraced what was troubling you, then it no longer has a hold on you. You will experience freedom and know that this particular pattern is leaving your life for good. This is the dismantling of the victim pattern.[11]

BJ shared an example of the process. She cited the Clint Eastwood comment I mentioned in chapter 1 about dealing with aging: "Don't let the old man in." While Eastwood meant just that, interestingly, BJ has a different perspective. She referred to the Allow, Accept, and Embrace technique of Gene Keys and recommended allowing the old woman in. Why? As BJ states, "Because she is older, perhaps wiser, and may have something to teach me." So, allow her in, over time accept her, and eventually embrace her, thereby performing a complete transformation.

This philosophy and technique can be used for all of life's personal challenges. BJ said, "This technique has been the biggest gift I've been given to identify my life purpose. My whole life I had been in a fighting stance. Fighting everybody—my mother, others, even myself. I now look at life and myself with loving eyes and embrace all that is." BJ recommends being gracious with your aging. She has softened. She doesn't need to fight herself anymore.

BJ realized the importance of purpose at her mother's deathbed. The need for purpose in our lives is one of the defining characteristics of human beings. Without purpose we are more vulnerable to boredom, anxiety, and depression. Having a purpose can provide a powerful positive effect. Purpose can enhance our self-esteem, our self-confidence. Each morning on waking you are more focused, knowing you're ready to make each day count.

There are several techniques for stilling the fluctuations of the mind and going inward for self-exploration of your purpose. Some include yoga, meditation, mindfulness, tai chi, and qigong. Another process is explored in Richard Rudd's book *The Art of Contemplation*. Rudd asserts that the real power of contemplation versus meditation or mindfulness is that it turns into decisive action that can bring about changes in our lives.[12] Additional information on contemplation is included in the Resources section at the end of this book.

The power of purpose is demonstrated in Victor Frankl's book *Man's Search for Meaning*, in which he describes his experiences in concentration camps during World War II. He observed that the inmates who were most likely to survive were those who felt they had a goal or a purpose. While Frankl attempted to reconstruct a manuscript he had lost, others held on to a vision of their future with loved ones once they were free.[13]

Studies show that having a purpose in life is not just enjoyable. It can make us healthier and more resilient and can even affect our mortality. Researchers at the University of Michigan's Department of Public Health identified strong evidence that associates life purpose and mortality.

In their study, participants fifty and older with the lowest life purpose had a 2.4-fold increased risk of death compared to those with the highest life purpose.[14]

A recent Stanford University study, "Purpose in the Encore Years," aimed to better understand the nature and implications of purpose for older adults so that professionals and organizations can better serve this population. Highlights of the findings of the nearly 1,200 survey responses indicated that 31% of older adults in the United States place a high priority on purpose and beyond-the-self goals. Their commitments are central to their identity and sense of meaning in life. The majority of respondents who indicated they were purposeful share a sense of positivity—joy, hopefulness, and optimism—in their lives.[15]

Part of making every day count is having a reason for getting up in the morning, a purpose. Interestingly, there is a Japanese concept known as "Ikigai" that focuses specifically on accomplishing this task. Additional information on this approach to living a more purposeful life is included in the Resources section at the end of this book.

Purpose can be defined in many ways. Some people find purpose in their jobs or special projects. Others find purpose in raising their children or being involved in their grandchildren's lives. Perhaps it's being of service to others as a volunteer. Or it could be a hobby or a passion. Having a strong purpose can have a positive effect on you and prevent negativity from creeping in. And it doesn't have to be a purpose with a capital "P." Just a purpose for you to get up every morning and make every day count.

PLANNING

"A goal without a plan is just a wish."
~ **Antoine de Saint-Exupery, author,** *The Little Prince*

By no means do I plan (pun intended) to provide a methodology for goal setting and planning in this section. But I have found that goals are but lofty dreams until we implement a plan of action to accomplish them. You might need to modify or alter a plan along the way, but that's part of the process. If there comes a time when you become overwhelmed or daunted by a task or project, never fear. As a dear friend has shared many times, when we're looking at what may be an unattainable or monumental undertaking, think of how one eats an elephant. One bite at a time. Wise advice that I have used many times.

If planning doesn't come naturally to you and you aren't sure where to start, consider the SMART system of planning as follows:

- Set a very **specific** goal.
- Determine a way to **measure** progress.
- Make sure the goal is **achievable.**
- Make sure it's **realistic.**
- Set a **time** commitment.

There are many ways to plan an intentional life, so find one that works for you. Following are examples of the planning process used by some of the Incliners that may inspire you.

Darlene: An Amazing Plan

Darlene's husband, John, often cites the fact that they were married in a hurricane in Aruba over twenty years ago and they are still living in one. What does he mean by this? If you were to meet Darlene, you'd understand the metaphor immediately. Darlene is one of the most purposeful and energetic people I have ever met. She had a successful career in global project management with IBM for over thirty years, and she used her innate ability to set goals and create plans for their successful completion. Darlene attacks every challenge in her life with energy and enthusiasm. And a sense of grace. She is always thoughtful of others' needs, often before her own. All of this helped her to reinvent herself at sixty.

She had a dream to be a motivational speaker so she could support women in following their dreams. Darlene worked diligently with a speaking coach and, when her new craft was honed, she started reaching out for speaking engagements. Today she is a nationally sought-after motivational speaker.

Four years ago, Darlene kicked up her goal aspirations with a bolder dream. She wanted to create a forum for fabulous, talented, and high-achieving women that are focused on supporting, inspiring, and motivating each other to have a bigger impact on the world. The Amazing Women Alliance was born. The members are all about "paying it forward" and providing an environment that helps everyone grow and reach their goals.[16] Today, at sixty-eight, Darlene's Amazing Women Alliance has a membership of 1,700+ women. Over ninety of them have graduated from her six-month Amazing Women Leaders program. The program helps women who want to enhance and grow their confidence and leadership skills, and achieve greater results, both professionally and personally.

So how has Darlene achieved this monumental accomplishment?

"I have to set reasonable and realistic goals. I need to be realistic with who I am and what I'm going to do. My goals are ever changing. They are not exactly what I thought they would be a few years ago. So, I make adjustments. In setting goals, I identify the steps to get there. That's where a plan comes in. Even though I might not stay on that plan, I need to know where I think I'm going, so for me that's my best way to get there. I have to keep my intentions and focus on my goal so there is as little distraction as possible."

There's no stopping this amazing woman who still lives life in a hurricane. She embraces climbing the hill and Inclining with gusto.

Judy: Intentional Retirement

When Judy was considering retiring from her position as a longtime educator and president of Fielding Graduate University, she applied the technique of intention that was used with great success at Fielding to her retirement planning. She entitled her process "intentional retirement" and continues to use it today at eighty-two. Judy strives to live with "intentionality"—being deliberate and purposeful. As a result, Judy is intentionally aging well with dignity, love, joy, and contribution. She lives authentically in her retirement. She also strives to be a positive role model for those she loves.

Her specific plan to live intentionally includes the following:

1. Strive to recognize that each of us can only be responsible for ourselves. We should not tell others what to do.
2. Only relate to giving, loving, positive family and friends. Try to forgive any slight.
3. Try to live joyfully and lovingly employ humor wherever possible.
4. Try to have one special thing to look forward to every day.
5. Listen carefully to others to truly understand.
6. Learn to say "No" and limit your community contributions to activities you truly love to do.

Every Sunday evening, Judy opens her "plan" book and outlines what her plans are for the coming week.

Judy is living with "intention." Intention is "a thing intended, an aim or plan." Judy's plan embraces both. She takes deliberate action to ensure she continues to live a meaningful and purposeful life.

Kristin: The Quintessential Planner

Kristin has the foresight to realize that we are living longer and she needs to start planning for what she wants her future to look like. She needs to ignore society's negative connotation about aging and not let it pull her down.

At forty-seven, Kristin's effervescent personality keeps on shining. She continues her successful career as a human resource director with great pride. A large part of her success, both personally and professionally, can be attributed to the fact that she is a quintessential planner, a trait that lends itself beautifully to planning her future so she can live a life of continuous Incline.

How does Kristin feel about the social perception that aging is all decline? She challenges society's ideas about what it means to age. Why? Because she sees so many wonderful examples of what people are doing in their seventies, eighties, nineties, and hundreds to continue to live meaningful and purposeful lives. She's changing her previous mindset and is now embracing that age is just a number. Kristin maintains, "I need to continue to show up every day, participate, and be engaged in my life. I'm starting to plan now. I'm not waiting until I retire."

To overcome the negative connotation of aging, Kristin has ceased her own negative self-talk. Kristin has taken the attitude of "Why am I complaining? Living to be older is a gift, and I need to take advantage of it and appreciate it rather than blame everything on aging. But I need to remember that just because I'm older doesn't mean I'm losing things. I've been gaining experience. I've been gaining wisdom. I need to appreciate that time is a gift."

Kristin has always been very focused on her career and work. However, she is now realizing she needs to take time to develop some hobbies and personal activities to take with her into her future, and she is working on that aspect.

And Kristin's future looks bright indeed. She has embraced the concept of Incline and is continuing to climb the hill.

While having a plan in place is wise advice, it's also important to anticipate what could go wrong. As Murphy's law points out, anything that can go wrong, will. As part of your planning process, implement a contingency or back-up plan. If you have a "Plan B," you won't be so easily derailed in the successful completion of your goal if something goes awry.

I invite you to celebrate joy every day. We are born with joy. It's inherently part of our makeup. As children, we look at life with eyes agog with joy. As we age and become adults, society tries to impose restrictions on us that squelch that joy. Let's return to the joyful spirit of our inner child.

Practice gratitude, which leads to being more resilient towards life challenges that you may encounter. Identify your purpose—either large P or little p—and plan your days to make every one of them count!

Review the tips and techniques in the Resources section at the end of this book. Hopefully, there is one that will tickle your fancy and titillate your interest or curiosity.

PERSONAL REFLECTIONS

1. How can you make every day count?
   Consider Judy's Intentional Retirement plan as a starting point.

2. How grateful are you?
   Take the Gratitude Quiz located in the Resources section at the end of this book and then consider implementing Angela's 3 Good Things practice, Carolyn's blessing and gift journal, or scheduling time with your "joy buddy."

3. What is one of your current goals?
   Consider creating a plan to achieve it using the SMART method.

CHAPTER 3

THE POWER OF PLAY

Ramona: The Waltz of the Flowers

What are your recollections of "play" as a child? What playful activities brought you the most joy? The ones that I bring easily to mind are somersaults on the lawn and lying in the grass watching the clouds sail by, imagining what animals they represent. But the one that's always at the forefront of my mind is the "Waltz of the Flowers." To this day, when I think of this beautiful music by Tchaikovsky from the Nutcracker, I can hear the music. I can feel a smile forming on my face and joy filling my heart. I dance as if no one is watching me. What a gift! That's the power of play!

Have you ever conducted a symphony of flowers as you danced in a garden?

We lived at 1 Douglas Crescent on Sea Island, near Vancouver, British Columbia, and I was in Miss Logan's Grade 2 class. One day she presented her students with a delightful exercise. She urged us to close our eyes and listen to the music she was about to play and imagine different flowers waltzing. When the music was over, she instructed us to use our crayons to draw the flowers we'd envisioned. Later that week I took it a step farther. I assembled my doll collection in my mother's garden and conducted my creation of an orchestra of flowers. Daffodils and jonquils served as wood and brass instruments, roses were the strings, and daisies were the percussion section. I danced around the garden with my dolls to the musical strains of the "Waltz of the Flowers" that still resonated in my head.

I was just playing with no purpose in mind other than for the sheer enjoyment of it. And I can reawaken that memory and relive it whenever I want—even today. While that sense of joyful play alluded me for many years, I have now regained that sense of freedom through the Nia Technique of dance that is featured later in this chapter.

As we grow older, we're conditioned by society to put aside "childish" games and take on the mantle of more serious adult responsibilities. Haven't we all been told to "act your age" when we were just having a bit of "playful" fun? What have we lost by giving up our ability to be spontaneous in our activities?

I propose we can return to that state of mind, which still resides inside all of us. It just needs to be reidentified. How is this done?

Recently I became fascinated with the concept of play when I was introduced to Stuart Brown's book *Play: How it Shapes the Brain, Opens the Imagination, and Invigorates the Soul.* Brown states, "Neuroscientists, biologists, psychologists, social scientists, and researchers now know that play is a profound biological process. It has evolved in many animal species to promote survival. But for human beings, play lies at the core of creativity and innovation."[1] He identified seven **properties of play**:

1. **Apparently purposeless:** done for its own sake
2. **Voluntary:** not required by duty
3. **Inherent attraction:** it's fun. It makes you feel good.
4. **Freedom from time:** when fully engaged, lose track of time
5. **Diminished consciousness of self:** we stop worrying about whether we look good or awkward, smart, or stupid. When we play, we are fully in the moment, experiencing what psychologist Mihaly Csikszentmihalyi calls "flow"[2] (which will be reviewed in greater detail later in this chapter).
6. **Improvisational potential:** we aren't locked into a rigid way of doing things. We're open to serendipity, to chance.

7. **Continuation desire:** we desire to keep doing it. And when it's over, we want to do it again and again.[3]

Reviewing these properties, I can check off each one relative to my experience with the "Waltz of the Flowers." Today, having reidentified and regained the freedom to play, I have found in the play of dance that I can once again check off all the boxes.

Play can be experienced in many forms—writing, drawing, painting, playing an instrument, learning salsa or tango, taking drama lessons, or playing pickleball. There are endless possibilities. Like many grandparents, my brother and sister-in-law, Raymond and Suzanne, attribute their youthful and joyful mindset to playing with their grandchildren, Ben and Matty. It helps them maintain a positive attitude towards aging.

Throughout her life, when my mother, Vera, was happy, she would kick up her heels and do a little dance just for the sheer joy of it! I always delighted in watching her as she generally was a little shy. But unwittingly her spirit knew how to express her happiness.

Brown contends that play is a state of mind rather than an activity. A study done in Okinawa, Japan, by the National Geographic Society revealed that engaging in activities like playing with young children was as important as diet and exercise in fostering the Okinawans' legendary longevity. Further, Brown maintains that "when we stop playing, we stop developing, and when that happens, the laws of entropy take over—things fall apart....When we stop playing, we start dying."[4]

Another advantage of play is the impact it has on our ability to be creative. Research studies conducted by Brian Sutton-Smith, a renowned play theorist, have shown that play-like activities put us into a psychological state where it's okay to fail. This allows us to freely explore the unknown. Play removes limits that otherwise constrain us and opens us up to exploring creatively.[5]

Interestingly, one of Brown's studies was a review of the role of play in childhood and adulthood and how it affects life course. He studied murderers in Texas prisons and found that "the absence of play in their childhood was as important as any other single factor in predicting their crimes." In addition, he documented abused kids at risk for antisocial behavior. Their predilection for violence was diminished through play.[6]

Brown contends that "play is the essence of freedom."[7] I now welcome a spirit of play, of childlike curiosity and delight, into my daily activities. Give yourself permission to play. You will free yourself from fear. It's time to remove yourself from the serious aspects of daily living and let loose. I guarantee that when you play, you'll smile and laugh more—both of which are good for the soul.

Lee: Keep the Inner Child Alive

Lee was previously introduced in "Turning Her Thinking Upside Down." When people ask her why she seems so happy and finds it so easy to laugh, she tells them, "My inner child is working overtime!" That belief has been with her for her entire adult life. Many times throughout the years, friends and relatives have remarked to her, in a not-so-kindly manner: "Lee, you're the biggest kid I know! Aren't you ever going to grow up?" Lee shared, "They're all dead now and I'm still here."

Now ninety-five, that "kid" or inner child has totally influenced Lee's thinking and her perception of life for the better. She can't believe she's been here so long! She can't believe she's had such a great life! When people started asking her how she's managed to live this long, she tried to explain her way of thinking. First, her inner child always has been alive and active. Then she was blessed with a loving, optimistic father who introduced her to humor and storytelling. He taught her to "love her life, love God, love people" and to believe in herself. Her mother, a good woman, pronounced herself "old" at sixty and, though she lived to age ninety-eight, was a total pessimist. Lee was not what she'd had in mind for a daughter. She did not know what to do with this child who was too loud, too full of fun, too optimistic. Lee thinks her mother is responsible for her being so hard-headed and determined.

Lee was very lucky to have a wonderful mentor from age thirty-four until her seventies. She taught her to pick herself up, brush herself off, and get on with her life when she was hurting so deeply. "Mama" Dodge was a perfect role model for thinking young and never growing old. She lived to be 100 years young. Lee can definitely testify: "Loving people and being a good active friend is paramount for happiness. And maintaining an 'attitude of gratitude' is included in that advice."

Lee's mantra is: "Keep your mind on what you want and off what you don't want. It works." Keep your inner child alive always—with curiosity, inspiration, laughter, and learning. While we have only limited control over what happens to us in life, we have 100% control over how we react. Therefore, older people who have learned to keep their sense of humor, think positively, and remain active, and who genuinely care about other people, continue to learn, and are interested in life in general truly are "young at heart" forever and die young even at 110.

Lee had a very interesting and successful career. She now spends a lot of time with her young friends (forties to eighties) going out to lunch, the movies, and theater. Compared to those seniors who are alert and active at 103 and older, Lee reports she is just a novice at this mature stage of her life, and she continues to keep her inner child alive.

This is strong testimony for maintaining a youthful attitude. I invite you to reconnect with your inner child and find an activity that gives you the freedom to reunite with your inner joy.

MOVEMENT

"Movement is the song of the body."

~ **Vanda Scaramella, yoga pioneer**

Amanda: Movement is Medicine

Amanda is the owner of MalaMotion, and her business motto is appropriately "movement is medicine."[8] She is a dancer and teacher and her repertoire includes dance, Pilates, yoga, and Gyrotonic. Amanda maintains, "Movement changed my life. I am positively a better mother, friend, daughter, teacher, and human being because of it."

Amanda brings such joy and creativity to movement. The knowledge and energy she brings to all her classes is seemingly endless. She has a deep understanding of the body, movement, and the value of health and fitness. And for her students, she delivers results.

Amanda was a gawky, ridiculously awkward tween and teen. Dance was her saving grace. It was what protected her heart when she encountered teasing, bullying, and body shaming. Movement and her relationship to it gave her hope to move forward as she developed a professional career performing in many different genres and types of venues for the better part of two amazing decades. That love of movement transformed into sharing the incredible techniques she now practices and teaches at age forty-five.

When asked if aging negatively impacts her, Amanda responded, "It enters my thinking every day, as I have two negatively aging parents who were previously very active. I can see in my father's body and sense of expression a surrender. It makes me livid." She has clients who are older and yet they are physically better than her parents, an illustration of what attitude and movement can do.

Amanda emphasizes to her students that proprioception is integral to movement of any sort and we should do activities daily to improve it. Proprioception is the sense through which we perceive the position and movement of our body, including our sense of equilibrium and balance. To put it simply, proprioception tells the body where it is in space. It's important to the brain, as it plays a big role in self-regulation, coordination, posture, body awareness, the ability to focus, and speech.

Proprioception is often referred to as our sixth sense. This sixth sense enables us to control the movements we make and provides us with the ability to understand ourselves moving in space.[9]

As Amanda elaborates, "When you know what a movement is doing inside your body anatomically and physiologically, your sense of movement and sense of your body as a whole grows. In turn, your understanding of proprioception becomes greater. And on a much more basic level, how our body relates to the space we're in."

Understanding and being in your body—what does that mean? Being in your body means more than just on a physical level, but also on an emotional and spiritual level. And, as Amanda contends, "Those three things combined gives us such an understanding in our daily lives of what we need physically, what we need spiritually. So proprioception can be this amazing catapult toward really feeling like you're in your home, which is your body, which is your self."

When Amanda teaches someone who hasn't had any movement background about proprioception, she gets them to really home in on what they do every day. We all brush our teeth, we all brush our hair, we all get in the car. Those are mundane activities and movements that our body does innately. So slow down a minute. Sit in your car. Note the pressure of your feet into the floor. How does that relate to your pelvis? When you brush your teeth, be more aware. Break down the basic movements we all perform every day into baby steps. Practice how to verbalize them. Write a journal about your movements. Become more aware of your body and how it interrelates to other parts, and your proprioception will grow from there.

Another advantage of being aware of your proprioception is that physical activity programs help maintain mobility. Researchers for Lifestyle Interventions and Independence for Elders (LIFE) conducted a study of more than 1,600 sedentary men and women at risk for disability. At the end of the study, the risk of major mobility disability for the group that had been assigned to a physical program was reduced by 18%.[10]

Amanda recommends exposing yourself to many different activities. When we engage in a physical activity every day, it wears into the neurotransmitters in our brains like a river. Over time, a natural riverbed-like path is produced in our brain and this activity no longer challenges us. But when we switch our activities around and add different physical processes, we challenge our brain and it becomes more resilient.

Personally, I agree with Amanda that it's advantageous to incorporate a variety of physical activities into one's wellness toolkit. In addition to attending regular yoga classes and having a home practice, I cycle with a stationary bike. I regularly attend Pilates classes and I've sampled tai chi and qigong. But, as mentioned earlier, it was Nia that was truly mind changing for me.

•

DANCE

"Dance is the hidden language of the soul."
~ Martha Graham, American modern dancer and choreographer

Julie: In the Flow with Nia

When Julie steps onto the dance floor, she lights up the room. She has the unique gift of combining movement and music to create magic when she teaches the Nia Technique of dance to her students.

Julie started dancing at the age of three. Dance has been a strong influence and pull in her life from that very young age. It is essential to the woman she is today. "One of the things I credit dance for in my life is that it was my sanity and my survival. I grew up in a home that was filled with fear. So to be able to daily go to dance class and seasonally put myself up on a stage in front of people were life-giving experiences."

As a young teenager, when her father asked her what she was going to do with her life, how she was going to make a living, she immediately responded, "I'm going to be a dance teacher." He very succinctly told her that she was going to need to figure something else out as that wasn't going to sustain her. While it was a huge disappointment for Julie, she accepted her father's advice.

After working in the corporate world for over two decades, Julie quit. As she says, "The work was diminishing me. I didn't have any self-growth tools or practices. Granted, I had enriching experiences with friends and family, but those were sort of outward experiences as opposed to inward experiences."

And then Julie stepped into a workshop called Revitalize and Energize in 2005. The magic of the moment was entrusting that she could step into this new year and her path would reveal itself. And Julie shared, "Doggone it, but they had a Nia class in that workshop. And I saw myself so very clearly in the front of the room teaching. In an instant I realized that was my foot back into dance."

Today, over fifteen years later, at fifty-seven, Julie inspires self-healing for others through movement and somatic education. Her teaching and facilitation experiences are sourced from Nia Techniques, Sun style tai chi, and other somatic mind-body education practices. Curiosity fuels her desire to foster conscious connections one on one or between groups from five to fifty.

"Becoming a Nia teacher created a big learning curve for me. It entailed learning about Nia, my body, and myself. But I realized I could become aware of my body, my emotions, and my spirit." She added, "And though they make a whole and they're impossible to dissect into parts, I can focus on those three. I can consider these components individually and learn more about myself and even find imbalances. And that imbalance is around functionality. Am I in the flow? Is my body still fluid or have I become rigid? And is it a rigid body that leads to a rigid mind that leads to a rigid heart? Or is it a rigid heart that leads to a rigid mind? They are certainly intertwined, but then how do I begin to break that up?"

For Julie it was Nia. "It's been fascinating for me to consider that flexibility and strength are physical characteristics and they're mental qualities and they're emotional qualities and that they can help me be the best me. That's the spirit part to it."

Nia has been a tremendous tool for Julie to learn more about herself. And, as Julie maintains, "Movement in everyday life is really a dance." So, let's join Julie and get "in the flow with Nia."

Flow

Have you ever been so absorbed in an activity that you literally lost track of time? All forms of play, including dancing, can create this sensation. Inherently, they all involve a sense of a free-flowing movement that provides a feeling of freedom, timelessness, and joy. In his book *Flow: The Psychology of Optimal Experience,* Mihaly Csikszentmihalyi outlines his theory that people are happiest when they are in a state of "flow." So, what is flow? Csikszentmihalyi defines it as "a state of concentration or complete absorption with an activity...that nothing else seems to matter."[11] In other words, you are in the zone or in the groove. Or, as Csikszentmihalyi described, "The positive aspects of human experience—joy, creativity, the process of total involvement with life I call *flow.*"[12]

Flow can be experienced in any activity. However, as Csikszentmihalyi contends, to be able to experience true flow, one must (1) have clear goals to strive for; (2) become immersed in the activity; (3) pay attention to what is happening (concentrate); and (4) learn to enjoy the immediate experience.[13]

While I have never been athletic, several decades ago I realized I needed to incorporate some fitness activities into my life for my physical and mental well-being. In addition to regular indoor cycling, I began practicing yoga and it's become part of my life. The benefits of yoga are numerous, including increased flexibility; increased muscle strength and tone; improved respiration, energy, and vitality; cardio and circulatory health; and protection from injury. Practicing yoga also provides an opportunity to experience mind-fulness. While there are several systems of yoga, the one I prefer and practice regularly is Iyengar. I've always enjoyed the structure of the series of linear poses involved in the practice. But a few years ago, I was looking for something new to add to my wellness toolkit, since I knew the benefits of participating in a variety of physical activities. I wanted something that would be more fluid in nature. And then I was introduced to Nia.

Nia is a holistic exercise approach that combines classic movement forms from the healing arts (including yoga), martial arts, and dance arts. It is truly a total mind, body, spirit celebration. As the developers of Nia, Debbie and Carlos Rosas indicate in their book *The Nia Technique: The High-Powered Energizing Workout That Gives You a New Body and a New Life*, "Nia is like chocolate. You can't describe it. You must taste it. It's pure joy!" As Debbie and Carlos assert, "The joy of movement is the secret of fitness. To feel good enough to last a lifetime, an exercise regimen must satisfy the heart and soul." [14]

In case you're wondering what the acronym "Nia" rep-resents, it has evolved over time since Nia was created in the mid-1980s. From Non-Impact Aerobics to Neuromuscular Integrative Action, it then progressed to the Swahili word for "with purpose." Currently, Nia means "Now I Am." I like this acronym. I can relate to it. When I dance, yes, Now I Am—here in the present moment, free to be myself, free to be in the flow, and free to experience pure joy.

The experience of this low-impact aerobic activity leaves me feeling buoyant, joyful. I lose myself in the music. There is a sense of freedom in letting yourself go. While there is a choreographed routine, you can still be spontaneous with your version. And there is no wrong step. Freedom of body and freedom of mind. I believe that adding the practice of Nia to my wellness toolkit has been one of the best gifts I have ever given myself. From me to me with lots of love.

For me Nia has been transformational—both physiologically and psychologically. That is, for my body and for my mind. Physically, my body is more relaxed and resilient. Mentally, my mind is more focused and resilient. The fluidity of movement allows me to regain that sense of freedom I experienced as a child when playing. I am now playing once again in Nia classes. And I carry that sense of joy I experience in class with me as I step off the dance floor and into my day.

Interestingly, neuroscientists have identified the best exercise for slowing down the aging process. And it's fun. Guess what it is? Yes. Dancing! According to a study published in the *Frontiers in Human Neuroscience Journal,* dancing slows down and even prevents the decline in the brain's ability to process mental and physical activity that comes with its natural aging process. Most physical activity slows down the brain's aging process. "But only dancing has proved to be effective when it comes to changes in behavior due to the noticeable improvements in balance."[15]

So, seek out your inner child and reclaim that sense of wonder, awe, and joy. Get in the flow! Get barefoot and join us on the dance floor!

Nancy SB: The Eternal Dancer

Nancy loved dancing from the time she could walk and move to music. She remembers dancing at a very young age to classical music in the living room of her parents' home long before she began taking dance lessons. Like many little girls, she had dreams of becoming a ballerina. By the time she was in high school, she was performing. Dance had become a part of her identity by then. She felt amazing when she danced, and she loved performing. As Nancy says, "Dance will always be a huge part of my identity. I can express myself more clearly in dance than I can verbally."

Nancy admits she was not a particularly great ballet dancer and after a year at the Royal Ballet School in London she decided to pursue modern dance. She has taught dance for over thirty-five years and loves sharing dance with her students. And she's passionate about mentoring young dancers and aspiring dance educators.

At the age of sixty-eight, Nancy is the lead instructor of Power for Parkinson's Dance. Power for Parkinson's is a nonprofit organization started in Austin, Texas, in 2013. Its mission is to improve the well-being of people diagnosed with Parkinson's disease. The fitness program has been developed using the most current research available regarding Parkinson's and exercise physiology. Since its inception, Power for Parkinson's has grown to provide free exercise, dance, and singing classes to over 300 people each week. Power for Parkinson's participants have an improved sense of well-being and report they are doing better physically, emotionally, and socially. Though Parkinson's can be difficult to deal with, adding exercise to one's routine is sure to improve overall health and a sense of well-being. People with Parkinson's disease reap physical, psychological, and social benefits from participating in the dance classes. [16]

Professional dance is a finite career, but says Nancy, "Working with people with disabilities or physical challenges has always been rewarding for me. I have always wanted to make a connection with dance. This is my retirement job. I want to be doing this until I can't walk anymore."

Bill: Motion is Lotion

I immediately knew it was Bill as he walked through the doorway of the coffee shop. He appeared to be in his eighties, as I'd been told, but while he walked with the assistance of a cane, there was a liveliness in his step and a twinkle in his eye.

Bill was diagnosed with Parkinson's disease several years ago when he started noticing a slight tremor in his hands. At first, he thought it was arthritis, but the doctor confirmed Parkinson's. How did he react? Bill has a very positive outlook on aging. So he took the diagnosis in stride and set out to learn how he could be proactive with the symptoms. The biggest challenge for individuals with Parkinson's disease is balance, so Bill regularly works with a physical therapist and incorporates balance exercises into his daily routine at home, focusing on straighter alignment in his body.

But it was a godsend for Bill when he learned of Power for Parkinson's three years ago. Bill stated, "When I walked into a room with other people who have Parkinson's disease, I felt like this was my community." He has been a student in Nancy SB's class for three years now. He uses a chair to aid with balance and while the dance routines don't necessarily focus on improving balance, they do help with coordination, range of motion, and strength. But most importantly, Bill says, "The dance classes are so much fun."

I mentioned to Bill that the sheer act of moving is healthy and related Amanda's mantra of "movement is medicine." He chuckled and said, "The Parkinson's disease mantra is 'motion is lotion.'" In other words, motion keeps your joints lubricated. He said after class he feels so energized, he goes home and does some of the dance moves again.

Bill is very happy with his life and emphasized that he really has blessings. He has enough money to live comfortably. He has a list of maladies as long as his arm, but he still considers himself blessed because "I don't have any major medical issues. And I don't suffer a lot of pain as many people with Parkinson's disease do. All of these blessings I attribute to my positive attitude."

He used to do a lot of dancing. That's how he met his current partner, Mary. While they no longer line dance, they are happy enjoying each other and living a blessed life with a positive attitude.

Bill's experience is a testament to the value of this program. I attended one of Nancy's classes to learn more about Power for Parkinson's, and it was a wonderful experience. The joy in the room as the participants danced was palpable. And the loving and nurturing way Nancy leads her classes and cares for her students was endearing.

I urge you to add a movement activity to your life, whatever form it takes. Better still, add several so there's some variety in your wellness toolkit.

CREATIVITY

"To practice any art, no matter how well or badly, is a way to make your soul grow."
~ **Kurt Vonnegut, author,** *Slaughterhouse-Five*

Tracy: Aging Creatively

Tracy personifies aging creatively. A quote she recently shared with me speaks to her positive mindset: "Attitude far more than your circumstances determines the quality of your life." I believe this positive mindset is due in part to Tracy weaving her passion for creative activities into her life.

As a former art teacher, Tracy continues her pursuit of her love of art. At seventy-nine, she is passionate about art in all forms. She is an accomplished artist who creates both sculptures and ceramic pottery of great beauty. She loves all things Japanese and has travelled to Japan many times to study Japanese culture and their forms of pottery and porcelain making.

Tracy created a piece of art to reflect the history of Black Americans. It's a road, a highway, the road she feels Black Americans have experienced with all its twists and turns. Tracy believes, "My life is a road, sometimes bumpy, sometimes with detours. That's the way I see it. I must make adjustments at every stage. At my current stage of Inclining, I continue to make adjustments."

Another creative pursuit for Tracy is her memory book, in which she includes information on everyone in her family who has passed away. She has their obituaries, death certificates, and facts on various other aspects of their lives. She's the go-to person in her family for historical information.

What is positive about aging to Tracy? She believes, "We learn wisdom, we learn patience, we become more spiritual, not necessarily religious. We must develop patience in order to get something done and to understand something. You're only going to get that as you age. So, there are lot of things we gain as we age but society doesn't promote that. They should.

"We have to reimagine and rethink our perception of aging. No matter what your age, as you age you get more like yourself. Just like a tree gets stronger and becomes more rooted in the ground, as we age, we become stronger. We are more and more like ourselves."

Tracy doesn't care for the term retirement. Many years ago, one of her professors said we should look at retirement as "redirection" and that's her perspective. When anyone says to Tracy, "You're retired," she responds, "No, I'm redirecting. Retirement is redirecting." It seems that Tracy is redirecting her life very creatively. Her artistic endeavors are keeping her young and vibrant. She is continuing to climb hills as she lives a life of Incline.

So many people think they are not creative. However, most have a passion for some subject to nurture their creative potential. Most of the Incliners in this book have hobbies, such as painting, sculpting, ceramic or pottery work, writing, crafting, and playing pickleball to name a few. Identify your passion and let your creative beast roar.

A tool to help your creative beast roar is Julie Cameron's book *It's Never Too Late to Begin Again*. It's a product of over twenty-five years of teaching. It's her attempt to answer, "What next?" for students who are embarking on their "second act."[17] This workbook is a twelve-week course for those who wish to expand their creativity. Several years ago, I completed the course. It was an amazing journey of continuing self-discovery. Additional information on the workshop is included in the Resources section at the end of this book.

Remember that sense of curiosity that was described in chapter 1? Albert Einstein said, "Creativity is intelligence having fun." Let's take a lesson from Einstein. Let your curiosity run rampant and creativity will be the reward.

Several years ago, I discovered the book *The Creative Age: Awakening Human Potential in the Second Half of Life* by Gene Cohen, MC, PhD. Dr. Cohen's philosophy of "creative aging" intrigued me and set me on an in-depth exploration of positive aging, as opposed to accepting the negative connotation of inevitable decline in vogue with society.

Cohen was a pioneer in the field of gerontology and his research of over thirty years began to put the misconceptions of decline to rest. It demonstrates that people in the second half of life can leverage their creativity to find a new sense of possibility. In Cohen's studies of aging people and in his work with them, four aspects of creativity stood out:

1. Creativity strengthens our morale in later life.
2. Creativity contributes to physical health as we age.
3. Creativity enriches relationships.
4. Creativity is our greatest legacy.[18]

Cohen founded the National Center for Creative Aging (NCCA). The center's mission is: "To ensure that older people have the ability to amplify their creative potential by leading and serving a diverse network of organizations and individuals to advance the creative aging field."[19] Over the years NCCA has partnered with organizations in most states in the US and several provinces in Canada to provide resources and creative programs to enrich the lives of older adults through arts education.

In order to reap the benefits, people need to continually develop and nurture their creativity. According to new research by psychologists at UC Berkeley, creativity tends to decline as we age. A series of experiments indicated that adults resorted to less creative thought processes than the children did. The research indicates that to be more creative, we need to teach ourselves to be more like kids. Rather than rushing through an activity, we need to take time to explore and discover as children do.[20]

As mentioned in the Introduction, as Inclined Elders continuing to climb the hill, we know there's no need to rush; it's not a race. We take one step at a time. In so doing, we have the benefit of pausing to smile at the waving wildflowers along the road. Apply that same attitude to your next adventure of curiosity.

As we age, many older adults fear an eventual loss of control over our lives and an inevitable dependency on others—be it family or care workers. Through Dr. Cohen's research, as contained in his 2006 publication *The Creativity and Aging Study,* he determined that "creative engagement promotes a sense of mastery and promotes social engagement—two key ingredients for healthy living."[21]

A sense of mastery creates a sense of control and leads to increased feelings of empowerment. This can influence individuals to reflect that if they performed well at one task, surely, they could master other activities. Creative activities, especially the arts, provide opportunities to experience a new sense of control or mastery. This sense of control has a positive effect on healthy aging. This is because the mind has an influence on the body.[22]

In addition, a growing number of studies have shown that social engagement in aging has a positive influence on health and reduced mortality. When the two dimensions of sense of control and social engagement are combined, it creates a highly sustainable healthy lifestyle. The practice of attending regular art classes is an excellent activity to accomplish this.[23]

In Dr. Cohen's study, the participants of the control group generally reported a decline in overall health. Conversely, those individuals who participated in the cultural group (i.e., art classes) reported an increase in overall health.[24] Yes, they were Incliners and continued to climb the hill.

PERSONAL REFLECTIONS

1. How can you get in touch with your "Inner Child" to relearn how to play?
   Consider watching children at play to see how effortlessly they do it. Or dance barefoot in your backyard. Let the grass tickle your toes and dance as if no one is watching. There is a sense of grounding to the earth when you are barefoot.

2. How do you get in touch with your "sixth" sense: proprioception?
   Review Amanda's suggested method.

3. What type of movement activity interests you?
   Consider a mindful walk in nature. Expand from there.

PART 2

GROWTH

*"Don't go through life,
grow through life."*

~ Eric Butterworth, author,
Discover the Power Within You

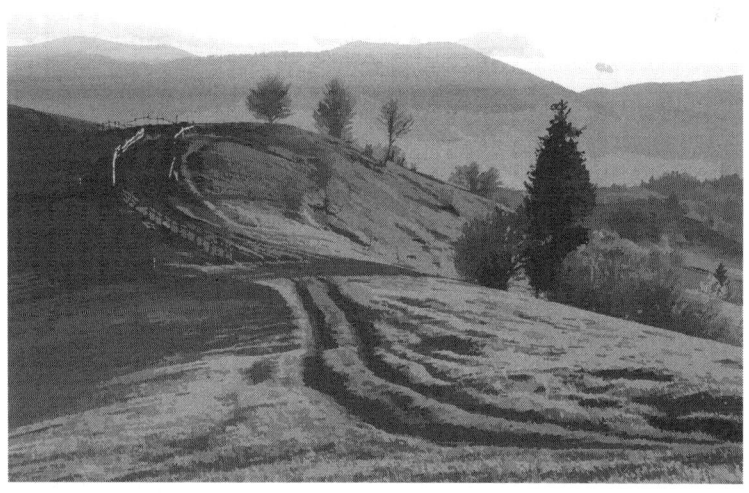

CHAPTER 4

EVER EVOLVING

"Connection is the energy that exists between people when they feel seen, heard, and valued; when they can give and receive without judgment; and when they derive sustenance and strength from the relationship."

~ **Dr. Brené Brown, author,** *Daring Greatly*

Dorie: Relationships Reign Supreme

The first things you notice about Dorie when you meet her are her engaging smile and then her exuberant personality. She was a teacher for many years, and then in 1990 she reinvented herself and became an award-winning realtor. She knew she could go a long distance with this career. At seventy-three she is still going strong. When people ask her when she is going to retire, she responds, "I want to continue to be useful and of service to others for a long time to come." What is the secret of her winning success? The relationships she makes with each and every client, many of whom become friends.

I'd known of Dorie and her successful track record for two decades but had never met her. When it came time for me to sell one home and purchase another, she was my go-to person—and she was amazing. We're now good friends.

One of the secrets of Dorie's success is her understanding that people want and need relationships in their lives. She has the following three quotes posted on her office computer and reviews them daily:

*"If you're always trying to be normal,
you will never know how amazing you can be."*
~ **Maya Angelou**

*"I've learned that people will forget what you said,
people will forget what you did, but people will never
forget how you made them feel."*
~ **Maya Angelou**

*"In the game of life, before you get anything out,
you must put something in."*
~ **Zig Ziglar**

Dorie lives by these credos and applies them in both her personal and professional life. She puts a great deal of love and care into every new relationship in the hope that people will derive benefit.

During her real estate career, Dorie's partner was her life partner, her husband, her best friend, her Gene. Many years ago, he had come across a poem regarding relationships. He so related to it that he decided that when the time came, he wanted it read at his funeral service. Recently, I was at Gene's service and heard the poem for the first time. It touched my heart. I have included excerpts of the poem below. The last two lines were added by Gene.

People Come into Your Life for a Reason, a Season, or a Lifetime

People come into your life for a reason,
a season, or a lifetime.
When you know which one it is, you will know
what to do for that person.

When someone is in your life for a REASON,
it is usually to meet a need you have expressed.
To aid you physically, emotionally, or spiritually.
Then without any wrongdoing on your part or
at an inconvenient time,
This person will say or do something to bring
the relationship to an end.

The prayer you sent up has been answered and
now it is time to move on.

Some people come into your life for a SEASON,
your turn has come to share, grow, or learn.
They bring you an experience of peace or make you laugh.
They may teach you something you have never done.
They usually give you an unbelievable amount of joy.
Believe it, it is real. But only for a season.

LIFETIME relationships teach you lifetime lessons.
Things you must build on in order to have a
solid emotional foundation.
Your job is to accept the lesson.
Love the person and put what you have learned to use in
all other relationships and areas of your life.
Thank you for being in my life,
Whether you were a reason, a season, or a lifetime.

~ Author Unknown

We all have people that come into our lives for a reason, a season, or a lifetime. Treasure and nurture them all for they are all precious gifts.

How can you build relationships beyond your family and your inner circle of friends? The answer is simple. Give generously of your attention, listen with your heart, and genuinely show that you care.

While Dorie and others like her inherently know the value of relationships, there is scientific evidence to support it. The author of *Aging Well,* George E. Vaillant, MD, worked as the longest-serving director of the now eighty-year study of human development, the Harvard Study. Vaillant describes human aging as a stone that is dropped into a pond. "It produces ever-expanding ripples, each older ripple encompassing but not obliterating, the circle emanating for the next ripple."[1]

Vaillant's study shows that:

"Close relationships, more than money or fame, are what keep people happy throughout their lives. Those ties protect people from life's discontents, help to delay mental and physical decline, and are better predictors of long and happy lives than social class, IQ, or even genes."[2]

For a good retirement, Vaillant recommends that people:

- Replace work friends with a social network
- Rediscover how to play
- Explore creativity
- Continue learning[3]

Humans are inherently social beings. The need for social connection doesn't fade with age. In fact, the need for social engagement and connectedness has profound implications for well-being as we age. When we are younger, school and work tend to provide the best opportunities to meet new people. So how do you make new connections as you age? Several good places to start include:

- **Volunteer:** select a cause or a professional group that's important to you
- **Religious Institution:** get involved with various activities or groups
- **Hobby:** whatever your area of interest, there is usually a club for people who share your passion. An online resource that matches people of like interests is www.meetup.com.

These are just a few. Use your imagination. The opportunities are limitless.

COMMUNITY

*"Alone, we can do so little;
together, we can do so much."*
~ **Helen Keller**

Christopher Peterson, one of the founders of Positive Psychology, states, "I can sum up Positive Psychology in just three words—Other People Matter. Period. Anything that builds relationships between and among people is going to make you happy."[4]

Peterson suggests that the "Other People Matter Mindset" includes:

- Identifying and appreciating the good in others
- Supporting them when they struggle
- Being present and giving others your attention
- Cheering their successes
- Knowing that your words and actions affect others[5]

David: A Good Man

When you meet David, the first things you notice about him are his warm smile and the whimsical wit he generously shares, especially during yoga class. Before retirement, he was a clinical social worker. On learning this about him I wasn't surprised, as he has a very caring nature.

David holds community as an integral component of his life and attributes it to his continuing happiness. Two of his top community groups are his church and the yoga studio where he regularly attends classes. He demonstrates wisdom as he selects groups that nurture both his mind and his body. At seventy-one, David continues to live an active life and has not experienced any noticeable aspect of negative stereotyping.

As an Incliner, David selects friends and acquaintances who share his positive mindset and attitude about aging. He doesn't know anyone who's ready for the rocking chair or has given up on life. He feels a little sad for those who have. How have they got themselves in this position and why have they given up? David doesn't think it's a question of age so much as attitude. He recommends connecting with people that have a similar mindset of continuous Incline.

For David, living life as an Incliner is not just about being self-aware, but putting effort into achieving that goal. It's trusting that other selected people will let him know when he's going off track. For David, it's his beloved wife, Kathy. David shared, "For me, self-awareness comes from reflection in prayer and in relationships. There are times I get frustrated, discouraged, down, whatever you want to call it or a combination of all of the above. Usually I just must step back and reflect. How did I get myself in this spot? What do I need to do to make it different?"

It's David's firm belief that the best way to overcome apathy, despair, and discouragement is through service. When you're actively serving others, you're less likely to get caught up in despair. He believes that we're only happy when we serve others. It's nothing to do with age. David thinks, "Sometimes we stumble upon that element as we get older, and so I get what it means. It's about learning how to be a more mature person. I know people in their sixties, seventies, eighties who are self-centered and guarded and apparently seeming to live a good life in some ways but, when you chip beneath the surface, they're not leading a life of service. They're leading a life of despair. Thus, service can bring meaning and purpose to your life."

David acknowledges that he always must challenge himself because his natural inclination is to pull back or be risk averse. So again, it goes back to being self-aware—noticing when you're becoming more risk averse and getting out of your comfort zone. Do more, not less. David thinks about that in terms of his friendships and his prayer life. "If I'm active in both, I'm less likely to hide in my cocoon. I need to push myself to get out there."

David tries to serve as a role model to younger people, such as his youth religious education class and members of his men's group. He often reflects, "Am I being a good man? Am I being a good Christian? I think if I'm doing those things—being self-aware, not being risk averse, living a life of service—the other stuff will follow."

So why is community important? As indicated in David's story, his church community forms the basis for his life as "a good man, a good Christian." He is very active with various church activities and projects that bring meaning and purpose to his life. I would say his faith and church work nurture his soul. His yoga community, of which we are both members, is a loving and caring group of individuals with a common interest. It not only nurtures his soul, but also his body, as he is practicing an exercise system that generates strength, flexibility, and overall well-being for body, mind, and spirit.

Community can provide a sense of belonging. Belonging to a group of like-minded people. It also creates a social and support network. And the need for social connection doesn't fade with age. Social engagement has profound implications for well-being, including self-esteem, physical and mental health, and overall life satisfaction. Older adults may suffer more than younger adults from a lack of social interaction.[6]

For many years, I served as a volunteer for a nonprofit organization in many capacities: volunteer, board member, and president. For me, it generated a sense of personal empowerment to serve others and gratitude for my ability to touch other people's lives in a positive way.

WellMed: A Center for Community

I recently had the pleasure and delight to become acquainted with many of the members of a local senior community center, WellMed. The moment I walked in the door and was greeted by the center manager, Valerie, I felt a sense of warm energy and happiness in the air. It radiated from everyone I saw.

As I was guided through the various activity areas, I was introduced to several members. What I witnessed were happy, engaged people. There was a group that enjoyed playing ping pong; another group was actively line dancing to the music of a local Western singer. Some were knitting or crocheting and chattering away. Others were practicing Power for Parkinson's. There was something for everyone. I glanced at the monthly calendar and the activities and projects seemed endless.

I had an opportunity to chat briefly with the "ping pong group" regarding their views on aging and what they enjoy about the center. Membership at the center starts at age sixty and the group I spoke with ranged in age from their sixties to their nineties. Their comments include the following:

- **Jimmy:** My wife has been ill. I got some home health for my wife and that's taken a bit of the burden off me. I'm getting back into doing some of the things I really enjoy like playing ping pong.
- **Gregory:** According to science, every cell in your body reproduces itself every seven years so medically you're never over seven years old. What can do a lot of damage is your belief system. My belief system is perfect because I have a positive attitude about aging.
- **John:** A friend introduced me to the center and right away I knew it was a community for me. It's just such a welcoming warm place. I enjoy the companionship. Apart from being active I think the most important thing is doing something that is meaningful to you. For me that involves doing a lot of volunteer work and giving to others. Trying to be kind, that's important. One other thing is having a sense of humor. And Gregory is a good model. Being able to laugh at yourself.
- **Uwe:** I think I'm lazy to be honest, but I do what my wife tells me to do. I try at least. We've been married for forty-six years and so far, so good. I get along with just about everybody. At the center we have parties, we dance, we laugh, we have fun. People need good

relationships with others to have a good life. We have that at WellMed.

Both David and the members of the WellMed Senior Center ping pong group understand and appreciate the value of community and that "other people matter."

LIFE COURSE

*"To create more positive results in your life,
replace 'if only' with 'next time.'"*

~ **Unknown**

Life Course versus Life Stages

Life Stages
During the twentieth century a three-stage model of life was prevalent: education, career, and then retirement.[7] But is anything really that simple? Indeed, in the 1950s, eminent psychologist Erik Erikson upped the number of stages to eight, while still maintaining that personality and life develop in a predetermined order. In his view, each stage built upon the previous one, an idea shared by Freud and many other scholars of the day.

One of the biggest problems I see with the life "stages" notion is the expectations and "rules" that go along with them: I'm an adult now, I should act grown up; I have a family, I should be responsible; I'm old so I should act my age and move to a retirement home. Isn't it time the idea that life revolves around a set of rigid, linear, predetermined stages—offered up by scholars and scientists and swallowed too readily by society—is examined more closely?

Well it has been. Thus, the evolution of the more fluid, resilient life course model, which you can choose to live by. You needn't accept that we're all doomed to move like automatons from one rigid life stage to another. You can choose to make changes in your life. Transition to new careers. Turn a passion into a new business or pastime. The Inclined Elders included later in this chapter did. They reinvented and rebranded themselves—sometimes more than once. You can too.

Life Course
Noted sociologist Glen H. Elder, Jr., defined life course as "a sequence of socially defined events and roles that individuals enact over time." These events and roles do not necessarily proceed in sequence, but rather constitute the total of the person's actual experience,[8] making it distinct from uniform life stages. Elder theorized the life course is based on five key principles:

- Life-span development
- Human agency (individual development)
- Historical time and geographic place (culture)
- Timing of decisions (adaptation)
- Linked lives (social integration)[9]

In addition, there is now a general shift in perspective among anthropologists interested in aging. Rather than a model that focuses exclusively on the lives of older adults, they are moving towards a more inclusive, multigenerational life course approach. They are recognizing that as individuals age, their lives unfold in conjunction with those of people of all different ages,[10] thus aligning with the "linked lives" principle of Elder's life course model.

The concept of the life course implies a more fluid, resilient model, distinctive from the rigid, uniform, predetermined concept of life stages. After all, there's been a reduction in the number of older adults banished to nursing homes or herded in droves to retirement communities because they're in the last "stage" of their lives. Thankfully, the focus is shifting to "aging in place," encouraging people to stay in their homes as long as it's practical, even creating "intergenerational" communities.

Andrea: Policewoman to Entrepreneur

A policewoman for eighteen years, at forty Andrea seesawed between continuing this secure career path until retirement or becoming an entrepreneur. While many people think most entrepreneurs tend to be young, this is not the case. In fact, 51% of small business owners are 50–88 years old, 33% are 35–49, and only 16% are thirty-five or younger.[11] Andrea realized she had a calling and was being led to make a change. So, she made the jump and did it. At forty-nine,

Andrea's business as a women's fitness and empowered living coach is thriving. But she emphasizes, "While I can be spontaneous in my decisions, I'm also a planner. There must be a balance." Andrea followed her heart but planned and prepared as much as she could before making the jump.

When making decisions, Andrea forgets about age and thinks about the things she wants to do and where she wants to go. As Andrea emphasized, "I just don't consider age, it's never been my focus. I don't allow it into my mind-set, my perception."

She maintains that it comes down to taking responsibility for where you want to be in your life. If you decide that at a certain age you want to be in an old folks' home and you believe you have limited choices, then that's the life you're going to live. Andrea thinks people forget they have a choice and they assume that this is what life is supposed to look like, so they think this is where they are supposed to be. Andrea challenges, "Why not buck the system of what 'aging' is supposed to be like and what stage you're supposed to be at. When you realize it truly is your choice—how you live and what living looks like—you can completely turn that around."

Inherently, Andrea courageously chose the more flexible and resilient life course model versus blindly accepting society's long-standing rigid, inflexible life stages version.

More and more older adults are returning to school or attending workshops to continue lifelong learning. Julie is an excellent example.

Julie: A Lifelong Learner

When Julie, the Nia teacher (chapter 3), asked herself, "As I age, how will I continue to Incline and grow?" her resounding response was, "Through education."

Julie certainly is living a life course instead of following society's life stages. Rather than continuing the linear path of life in the corporate world, in her forties she returned to her passion for dance and has been teaching ever since. For her, lifelong learning is a principle of living a more fluid, resilient life course.

For Julie, growing up and school were terrifying. Anything less than an A brought on some sort of a scolding or a talking to, an admonishment. So learning was never ever fun at all. When she graduated, she thought, "Thank God, I'm done with school. Let's move on from here. Let me just get out of here and do this thing called life."

Julie spent many years working and being in a career. But it never dawned on her that people could continue to learn. It took attending grief counseling after her husband's death for her to realize that people can continue to learn all through life. "So, this is 'lifelong learning.' I'm so glad to have overcome that misconception about learning. I've found learning again. Can I keep growing all the way through? Yes. And that's what I'm doing and that's what I model and that's what I'll continue to share with as many people as I can. I want to be part of a movement that dispels the fear around aging, getting older. Because fear is the emotion that came up for me. I don't want to be part of that negative aging thing."

In addition to her work as a somatic educator teaching Nia and tai chi, since 2009 Julie has served as a volunteer facilitator for a local nonprofit called Truth Be Told. She teaches creative writing and other subjects to incarcerated women. At fifty-seven, not only is Julie teaching selflessly to this community, but she continues to learn from them as this group of women are lifting each other higher by sharing their truths.

Through education Julie realized she could gain understanding, begin to help herself, and become happier. She could let go of things that she didn't have to hold onto. That's been a lengthy and continuing process for her. "I tend to sort of lean over when my chest is down, or my heart is down. In the past five or ten years I've been thinking, what is it going to be like to hold my heart up? It's different than holding my head up. To hold my head up was how I was at work. And then slowly I learned more about how to hold my heart up. Then it was easy. I was holding it up."

Julie recently posted a picture of a lifeline project on a social media site. A colleague she hadn't heard from in a while posted back asking if she was writing a book. Julie thought, "How fascinating that she would be interested in what I have to say. It didn't necessarily mean to me that was the universe's way of saying write a book. What felt groundbreaking to me was the AHHH, I'm holding myself back. And I didn't realize I was until somebody saw me differently than I see myself. That was a huge revelation."

As Doris Lessing, the winner of the 2007 Nobel Prize in Literature, asserts: "The great secret that all older people share is that you really haven't changed in seventy or eighty years. Your body changes, but you don't change at all." Thus, our core essence remains intact. Yes, we are all aging, but let's shift from a chronological mindset to one of an ageless "self" so we can continue to live our lives with purpose and enjoyment.

Let's not relinquish those things that brought us the most joy when we were younger: our dreams, our passions, our crazy ways of youth. The essence of who we are will always be with us. So let's just say "screw it" to the expectations of others. That's the legacy that life stages tend to deny those who fall into its trap. And, not surprisingly, it's taken the new worldview of the Boomers, together with our extended life span, to see the fallacy in that earlier thinking, at least when it comes to the sense that most people can enjoy a fully satisfying and meaningful life, regardless of age.

Perhaps it's time we dispelled a myth associated with aging—the supposed midlife crisis.

Midlife Crisis vs Middlescence

Midlife Crisis
Let's look at one of the biggest social constructs of all time: the "midlife crisis" is a term invented by the Canadian

psychoanalyst Elliott Jaques for a theory he presented to the British Psychoanalytical Society in London in 1957. He proposed that the period of midlife (then thirty-five, as average life expectancy was seventy) is ignited by the awareness that your life is halfway over, and death imminent. So, not surprisingly, the likes of you and I may be compelled to take measures to attempt to remain young.

When Jaques' paper was published in the *International Journal of Psychoanalysis* in 1965 under the title "Death and the Midlife Crisis," the idea jumped into the popular culture. The midlife crisis now became an inevitable part of life, not just some academic's theory. It morphed into the cliché of men in their thirties or forties purchasing a shiny new sportscar or fantasizing about vivacious younger women, while women opted for a face-lift and lusted after boy toys. Picture Marilyn Monroe in *Seven Year Itch* standing atop the subway grate with her white dress billowing around her while being ogled by her neighbor. Or Glenn Close in *Fatal Attraction*, boiling the pet rabbit because she was having issues getting her man.

The midlife crisis became woven into every aspect of the fiber of our culture—all based on a term invented for a theory. And the clichés persisted until the 1990s, when scientists and researchers began to reassess the validity of the concept of the midlife crisis and determined that it wasn't biologically induced, but just a social construct or theory. Yet, this sticky idea, so embedded into our youth-obsessed culture, persists even now.

Middlescence
Nonetheless, at midlife many adults pause to assess where they are now and what they have wanted to accomplish in their lives to this point—somewhat of a stocktaking. There can be a sense of disappointment if some life goals have not been accomplished yet. But the emphasis should be on "yet." Because rather than looking at this midpoint as a time of "crisis," it should be viewed as a time to assess, make changes if necessary, yet continue to Incline.

While the term midlife crisis denotes a period of unwelcome life changes and a signal for inevitable decline as we age, gerontologist Barbara Waxman proposes another theory. She feels it's time to change the perception of what it means to be an adult in midlife, what she calls "middlescence." It's a new stage, one that considers the demographic realities of an evolving world and rejects the negative norms of the past. Ms. Waxman defines "middlescence" as:

> A transitional period, between the ages of forty-five and sixty-four, marked by an increased desire to find or create greater meaning in one's life. Often accompanied by physical, social, and economic changes, it is a turning point from which adults continue to develop and grow. A life stage created by increased longevity patterns in the twenty-first century.[12]

Those adults who identify as "middlescents" in midlife are embracing the realization and certainty that they can continue to live a life of Incline.

Barbara Waxman created the Thriving Quiz, a tool to score yourself on the five essential areas for a successful midlife:

- Physical Well-being
- Rest and Renewal
- Attention and Focus
- Meaning and Purpose
- Time and Energy Management[13]

A link to the Thriving Quiz is located in the Resources section at the end of this book.

Interestingly, the U-Curve of Happiness, discussed later in this chapter, supports Ms. Waxman's theory of "middlescence" and the premise of *Inclined Elders.* While there is a downward dip in happiness levels during midlife, it increases upwards well into later life, signifying the continuation of Inclining.

Inclined Elders: Life Course—Reinventing and Rebranding

Unknowingly, most of the Incliners have accepted the more fluid, resilient life course model over the rigid inflexible life stages linear path because the life course model invites change. This reinvention or rebranding of oneself is very often used by individuals transitioning at various times in their lives. Lifelong learning is an integral part of these transitions. Many of the Incliners interviewed for this book have reinvented themselves:

- A high school English teacher for many years, Darryle always had a strong interest in the history of the Holocaust. She taught a unit on the Holocaust in her English classes. She then taught Holocaust classes at a local university. Darryle also leads Holocaust Educator Workshops. She has been instrumental in bringing Holocaust survivors to speak at various events, including Nobel Peace Prize winner Elie Wiesel. At seventy-five, Darryle continues to pursue her passion. She believes it is so important that future generations hear the story of the Holocaust. In doing this, Darryle hopes she can change the way people treat others who are different than themselves.
- Phyllis has reinvented herself many times over. Originally in finance, she then focused on communications and marketing, and eventually trained to become a chiropractor. Combining her experience in all these fields led her to develop a methodology to help children with dyslexia. At seventy-three, she continues her practice.
- In their late fifties, Fran and Bill left the corporate world of IBM to follow Bill's lifelong passion for photography. They started a business that specializes in producing and capturing beautiful and creative fashion, portrait, advertising, editorial, and event

photos, which involves intense planning, long hours, focus, and at times physical effort. Interestingly, at sixty-two and sixty-three, Fran and Bill frequently have more stamina than their much younger team members.

- Jim left a secure position in IT in his sixties to move to a small town where he joined the volunteer fire department. He then trained and became certified as an EMT (emergency medical technician) and now is director of the local food pantry. He went from work as a computer tech to fully embracing and supporting public service.

How were these Incliners able to make changes and reinvent and rebrand themselves? For some, like Darryle, it was a strong curiosity or interest in an area that they developed into something bigger. For Phyllis it was a matter of further education to reinvent herself and explore new opportunities. For all, an underlying common thread was a strong belief in being able to make the change, a commitment to lifelong learning, and taking a leap of faith, at times, to make the move. They used a hobby, a passion, further education, or a combination as leverage to make the move.

GENERATIVITY AND INTERGENERATIONAL LIVING

Tracy: Self-Segregation or Generativity?

Tracy (Aging Creatively, chapter 3) and her husband continue to live in their home and are very active with their family, friends, and community. They interact with people of all ages and are not interested in senior citizen communities. Tracy doesn't care for them because she thinks people who live in them self-segregate themselves. She believes it would be better for everyone emotionally, physically, and mentally if there were more places that include several generations.

"There needs to be an emphasis on a continuation of life. Young people witnessing old people getting older. The old people being influenced positively by young people. As you get older you must readjust to the new things in life. Some of the new things I feel young people would be sharper at and be able to teach their elders." Thus, a sharing of elder wisdom and youthful knowledge. A win-win relationship. Tracy would like to see more of an intergenerational approach.

Tracy and her husband understand the significance of several generations intermingling with each other. Inherently, they have embraced the concept of "generativity." The term generativity was coined by the psychoanalyst Erik Erikson and is defined as the "ability to transcend personal interests to provide care and concern for younger and older generations."[14] He suggested that in midlife we should be striving for generativity rather than stagnation. As humans we have a desire to satisfy this need for generativity, for generating good things and good people.[15]

Erikson concluded that, as we get older, we realize: "I am what survives me." Having children is the ultimate act of generativity, but giving birth can be experienced in so many other ways: creating a work of art, a recipe, a novel, a business. It can also refer to creating the very future itself through teaching, nursing, and volunteering at social institutions like community centers, churches, and schools. "What we generate moves into the future and provides for those coming after us. *I am what survives me.*" And in the process of this birthing, this creating, this generating, we are sharing these gifts with others and potentially interacting with multiple generations.[16]

Multigenerational or intergenerational living is defined as including two or more generations, such as grandparents and grandchildren, in one household. While the affordability of housing and other economic factors play a large role, there are other benefits such as easing the burden of childcare and reducing isolation for older adults. One of the biggest advantages is providing two-way learning and mentorship opportunities—"transmission of life wisdom to a younger person, and technology training for an older adult." That interaction across the generations helps us to nurture a cultural shift in how people think about age and aging.[17]

Unlike in the US, many countries are recognizing the benefits of intergenerational living and promoting and prioritizing this lifestyle.[18]

The Kampung Admiralty in Singapore is a large integrated living complex that opened in 2018. The focus of the development is residents' integration into the broader community. A childcare center is located alongside eldercare facilities. People that reside at Kampung have bought into the intergenerational vision and take full advantage of the facilities. Another example is Germany's multigeneration house program. Over 500 houses operating under the program are gathering hubs in communities throughout Germany. The houses create a "social space orientation" approach that provides a range of intergenerational offerings to each specific community.[19]

Marc Freedman, President, CEO, and founder of Encore.org believes, "The goal of later life isn't trying to stay young; it's to be there for those who actually are young." Encore.org aims to solve social problems by harnessing the experience of people in midlife and beyond through various programs and opportunities. Today, with more people in the US over fifty than under eighteen, a growing resource is available.[20]

So, how do we leverage a society that has more old people than young? In his book *How to Live Forever: The Enduring Power of Connecting the Generations,* Freedman presents his view that the generations can create a richness of life together that neither one can have alone. We can tap into this largely underused talent of older men and women to support the next generation, not only within families but in the broader community.[21] This is what he has been doing successfully for many years with programs such as Generation to Generation, which recruits adults over fifty to work with children to improve their prospects, and Experience Corps, a service program that engages people over fifty-five.

Christopher Peterson's succinct definition of Positive Psychology from earlier—"Other People Matter"—sums up the significance of this chapter. As humans, we are social beings that need the interaction and stimulation of others—connections and community with both young and older generations. We need to continue our love of learning, delve into our curiosity, and open our minds and hearts to a boundless vista of new adventures as we continue to Incline.

PERSONAL REFLECTIONS

1. What are some of your interests?
   Find groups that share your common interests. Or consider something new. Perhaps volunteering in your neighborhood. New relationships are sure to follow.

2. What are you doing, or what can you do, to continue your personal growth?
   Consider expanding on the interest you identified in chapter 1, question 2. Curiosity and lifelong learning go hand in hand.

CHAPTER 5

VENERATE NOT DENIGRATE

CULTURE

*"A nation's culture resides in the hearts
and in the soul of its people."*

~ **Mahatma Gandhi**

In 1871 Sir Edward Tylor, founder of cultural anthropology, defined culture as "that complex whole which includes knowledge, belief, art, morals, law, custom, and any other capabilities and habits acquired by man as a member of society." Tylor's focus on knowledge and belief as acquired— that is, *learned*—by members of a social group, continues to inform our sense of what culture is.[1] In turn, these learned behaviors are then shared with members of a group of people. While there are differing definitions of culture amongst anthropologists, most agree that culture has to do with those aspects of human awareness and activity that are derived from what we learn as members of a society.[2]

Culture is something that differentiates one society from another. It refers to the set of beliefs, practices, and learned behaviors passed on from one generation to another.[3] Put simply, it is the "way of life" of groups of people, the way they do things, and, more importantly, the attitudes of groups. This all indicates that individuals and groups have the ability to make choices about their attitudes.

Dora: Culture in Transition

In the Hispanic culture in which Dora grew up, the elders were considered the most important people in her family's lives. They were always looked up to. As they aged, somebody in the family brought them into their home to take care of them. "We took them everywhere we went. We did everything based on what Grandpa and Grandma thought we should do. Or what Mom and Dad thought we should do. That's just the culture I grew up in." Veneration for elders was woven into the fabric of everyday life. Reverence and respect for their wisdom was assumed.

But fast-forward to Dora raising her family. Because her extended family is no longer living near one another, that village concept isn't in place anymore. Her children are not growing up with the same cultural norms. As Dora considers, "I kind of step back sometimes and think about what that looks like now for my kids. I see my culture being diluted a little bit." In some ways she considers it positive because someone like her would not have been able to attend university a couple of generations ago. In her family she is one of six sisters. She is the only one, the first, with two college degrees. Dora concludes, "So it's just a whole different world from where I came from."

At forty-seven, Dora still venerates her grandparents and parents alike. And she has instilled this sense of respect for elders in her children. While her family may no longer be living in proximity, that ingrained cultural value of respect for elders is still there. And, of course, it's Dora's hope that it will continue to future generations of her family.

Let's compare some cultures that traditionally venerate their elders with our society that generally does not.

Global Aging and Cultural Transitions

In some cultures, such as in India and Japan, elders have traditionally been venerated and respected. Generally, it's not uncommon to have three generations living in one household. And yet even these cultures are seeing changes to cultural norms.

"The first decade of the twenty-first century has been marked by a dramatic interest and growing concern over an unprecedented human transformation, the global aging of human populations."[4]

Unprecedented changes are occurring worldwide as fertility rates decline and there is a significant increase in human longevity, with twenty to thirty years added to previous life spans for some. In former centuries, plotting populations by age group yielded a pyramid shape. In most societies the young, at the base, exceeded the old, at the tip. However, with global aging, pyramids have been morphing into rectangles. It's projected that as early as 2030 the percentage of Americans sixty-five and older could exceed the percentage that is younger than fifteen.[5] And this trend isn't just applicable to our society. It's manifesting globally.

So, as with Dora's cultural transition, this is occurring in other cultures worldwide, sometimes with positive implications and sometimes not. In many Asian countries, societies that were much more grounded in interdependence and family, this culture can no longer be maintained fully because of demographic and social change.

In India, the notion of lifelong intergenerational living is currently going through a major transformation.[6] While the majority of Indian elders, about 80%, continue to live in a multigenerational family setting, there has been a tremendous rise in the number of senior citizen care centers. Many older Indians feel that this shift from the traditional family model of adult children living with and caring for their aging parents is diluting respect for individual elders and their broader culture—their whole way of life.[7]

Interestingly, in response to a broad societal decline in family-based care and respect for elders, in 2007 the Indian government enacted legislation that stipulated children must support their parents or be subject to fines and potential imprisonment.[8] The Indian government amended many clauses of this legislation to ensure better care and maintenance for the senior citizens, including expanding the definition of "children" to include daughter-in-law and son-in-law.[9]

Japan is also experiencing challenges. The aging of Japan's population has progressed much faster than other developed countries. In 1990 the percentage of people sixty-five or older was slightly above 10%. As of 2015 it had jumped to 26.6%,[10] the highest in the world. It's projected that by 2060, 40% will be sixty-five and older.[11]

Traditionally, sons are expected to take care of their parents. To have three generations under one roof was once considered a symbol of happiness and fortune.[12] However, as with so many older adults, it is placing a burden on the family to care for their elders. This is increasing the potential for greater abuse of the elderly, including emotional or physical abuse and neglect. Japan took a stand to reverse the problem of elder abuse and in 2006 enacted the Elder Abuse Prevention Act to reduce incidents.[13] This has occurred in a nation that traditionally venerates their elders.

On a more positive note, no doubt we're all familiar with Dan Buettner's Blue Zone research. He teamed up with the National Geographic Society in 2004 and identified five regions around the world with the highest life expectancy, or with the highest proportions of people who reach age 100. (Incidentally, they are called Blue Zones because, when Buettner and his colleagues identified these areas on a map, they drew blue circles around them.) The most well-known of these Blue Zones is the Japanese island of Okinawa.

In most Blue Zone areas, senior care homes don't exist. A combination of family duty, community expectations, and genuine affection for elders keeps centenarians living with their families—creating an intergenerational lifestyle. Buettner and his team found nine common denominators of Blue Zone areas, primarily centered around diet and lifestyle. Blue Zones tend to be places where the culture emphasizes health and social well-being. These factors are all optimal for extremely long life expectancies.[14]

While the underlying value of veneration appears to continue to be interwoven into the culture of these Asian countries, global aging has had an impact on maintaining their cultural norms.

Western Society's Culture in Transition

While so many other societies continue to venerate their elders despite cultural challenges, Western society is a youth-centric culture that generally denigrate elders and looks negatively upon the entire concept of aging. The emphasis is placed on maintaining our youth. It's all about anti-aging. We see and hear it everywhere. There is a constant bombardment of late-night talk show hosts going on about the older age of presidential candidates and other political figures compared to positive views of elder states people in other countries. Makeup companies promote products that will make you look younger—by fighting aging.

Elders are viewed as senile and incompetent, decrepit, and over-the-hill. Aging is seen as a state of perpetual decline. Our entire society tells older people that they are useless, unwanted, and a burden. It tells younger people that getting old is bad and being old is worse.

Isn't it about time that we wake up as a society and understand and acknowledge the value of our elders? That rather than being a burden, they are contributing members of our society? Rather than old and decrepit, senile, and over-the-hill, many are continuing to have meaningful and purposeful lives and are thriving as they embrace an attitude of Incline. Let's promote a society that is more considerate of elders' needs, values their contributions, and doesn't dismiss them as irrelevant. Let's eliminate the "fear factor" in our society that aging and being old are bad. Because this "fear factor" has been manufactured by society. Just look around you at all of us fifty-, sixty-, seventy-, eighty-, and ninety-somethings that are still alive and well and having a heck of a good time living meaningful and purposeful lives. We can certainly debunk the myth that elders are a drain on society because we are useless, decrepit, and senile. That's just not the case. We're still productive members of society, whether we're working into our seventies and eighties, being childcare providers for grandchildren, sharing our wisdom and knowledge in service such as volunteering, or in other capacities.

Positivity and Happiness

Despite this negativity towards aging embedded in our culture, older people still tend to rate themselves happier than younger generations. Call it experience or perspective or wisdom—older people just seem to have an easier time coping with adversity and focusing on the good in their lives. Dr. Laura Carstensen, the founding director of the Stanford Center on Longevity, is one of the nation's leading thinkers on the social psychology of aging. Instead of finding that old people are grumpy or dotty, she has found that they are positive. She has termed this phenomenon the "positivity effect." Her research found that people tend to get happier as they get older. Such emotional positivity can impact the overall quality of life of older people, including the cognitive abilities of attention and memory.[15]

U-Curve of Happiness

Other scientific research also demonstrates that older people are happier. A relatively new branch of economics referred to as "happiness economics" proposes the "U-Curve of Happiness." Based on the findings from many global surveys, it appears that in our early years, our life satisfaction or happiness level is high. However, in midlife it takes a noticeable dip for the first couple of decades of adulthood and then increases again with age, thereby creating the "Happiness U-Curve."[16]

So how can we make sure this stays the case? By eliminating the negative stereotype of aging, that is, ageism. By continuing to live our lives as Incliners, thereby serving as role models to younger generations that aging is not the doom and gloom it's been hyped up to be. It can be a positive experience filled with new adventures and a sense of great joy.

Darlene: I'm Not My Grandmother!

When asked how she felt about the social reality of decline, Darlene (An Amazing Plan, chapter 2), commented, "It always has an impact on what people think aging looks like. I can't tell you how many people tell me I look much younger than I am. So, there's a stereotype of what older people should look like. And it has to do with the concept of decline. We must change that. Because we are very different from our grandmothers. We're very different from our mothers, but I think decline is a perception, that is, the social perception of decline."

Darlene doesn't envision herself sitting in the rocking chair at the old folks' home any time soon. She sees herself continuing to climb the hill. Thus, she's a natural Incliner. "But if we, as a society, don't have an attitude of Incline and if we don't look at aging differently, then we will end up in that rocker sooner than we want. I believe it's up to us to effect change with attitude and mindset."

People often tell Darlene that she's too old to have long hair. Her response is, "Why not? I don't understand that.

That's a perception that society has decided." She added, "Older women shouldn't look like teenagers. I certainly don't want to look like a teenager, but I don't want to look like I'm ninety years old either. Don't allow people to put you in that box that society wants you in." At sixty-eight, Darlene is becoming way more aware of her health and the things she needs to do to maintain it. What does Darlene do? "I keep my intention and my focus high to reduce distractions. That's my plan."

Darlene believes that one way to change the stereotype is to demonstrate that we're still living our lives with meaning and purpose as we age. We're setting an example. She said, "I think that's an awesome way to show others what we're doing and how we're doing it. And to show that it can be done. Just like I said earlier when I talked about my grandmother. I loved my grandmother, but my grandmother always seemed old to me. I seem older to my grandchildren but in a different way. They see me having a meaningful, purposeful life as I continue to Incline. I think that's the way to do it."

"If I were to rebrand aging, I would not put a number on it. Everyone must age in their own way. Just be yourself. Don't let someone else dictate what you should do or who you should be. If we do, that's when we start losing our ability to move forward and continue to Incline."

Darlene is the total opposite of the stereotypical grandmother.

Stereotyping

A stereotype is a mistaken idea or belief many people have about a thing or group that is based on how they look on the outside, which may be untrue or only partly true. Stereotyping is a type of prejudice because what is on the outside is a small part of who a person is on the inside. Ageism is prejudice against a particular age group—especially the elderly.

This ageism is often worse for older women than older men. There's a definite double standard. I recall the saying, "Men age like a fine wine, women age like a glass of milk." How horrifying is that? In our society, men with gray hair are usually referred to as distinguished while women are thought to just look old, even when such Hollywood celebrities as Diane Keaton and Jamie Lee Curtis have gone gray beautifully.[17] Yet many women continue to dye their hair, knowing that the first impression we make with someone new—what I refer to as a "Kodak moment"—can be negative.

Let's accept women's choices either way—to be gray or not, and other choices with respect to aging. Just celebrate the amazing, beautiful, wise women you are, and the inner light of who you are will shine through.

Historically there has been a prevalence of societal stereotyping of certain groups of people. We tend to label people based on very quick assessments. Society needs to address ageism in the same way it has addressed other "isms" such as racism and sexism. We need to take a stand and address ageism and the negative assumptions about older people.

You see it on greeting cards that represent old people as over-the-hill and sitting in the rocking chair on the front porch of the old folks' home. Age discrimination in employment is also very prevalent. With my background in human resources, I witnessed it firsthand. More mature people who were qualified candidates for a position many times would be passed over for younger ones. Subtle, but it was there, even if unspoken.

Nowadays people recognize that it's wrong to stereotype women or people of color. However, they don't see that ageism is the same thing. People don't even consider it a bad thing to do. We don't see it as injuring an individual or a group of people. But in stereotyping older people as decrepit, senile, and over-the-hill, and aging overall as a spiraling decline, we are placing limitations on older people. Open your eyes and look around at all the people you know who are in their sixties, seventies, eighties, and beyond. They are continuing to live meaningful, purposeful, active lives. Remember all the Inclined Elders whose stories are included in this book. They are living proof, and there are a lot more of us out there.

Following are some ways you can contribute to this overall change in perception—from a social perception of decline to one of continuing Incline.

- Change your mindset. Choose and embrace a positive attitude towards aging and stay active in ways that matter to you.

- Let go of outdated stereotypes about older adults.
- Be proud of your age and share it. As Miss Lee of "Keeping the Inner Child Alive" taught me, precede your age with "J-U-S-T"—for me, I'm currently "just 70."
- Keep the inner child alive.
- Don't allow people to put you in the box that society dictates for you.
- Demonstrate that you're still living your life with meaning and purpose, thus serving as a positive role model for younger generations.
- Plan to be intentional and focused about how you want to live your life as you age.
- Don't allow younger people to be dismissive towards you. Speak up, be heard. Turn that invisibility shroud to one of "Look at me. I'm here. And I'm proud of where I am."

Let's shift the mindset of society and people young and old who buy into society's negative connotation that aging is all about decline and being over-the-hill. Let's stop compartmentalizing age groups. Let's value the older population, celebrate our elders for all their contributions to society, for their value, their wisdom. And, above all, let's eliminate the "fear factor" that aging is all about decline. Because it's NOT! By embracing this positive attitude, we can change society's negative connotation and demonstrate that, as we age, we can continue to Incline.

WISDOM

"We are not provided with wisdom,
we must discover it for ourselves, after a journey
through the wilderness which no one can take for us,
and effort which no one can spare us."

~ Marcel Proust, French novelist

The Five Character Strengths of Wisdom

Theologians, philosophers, and others have attempted to define wisdom for thousands of years, including Socrates, Aristotle, Descartes, and Confucius. I rather like Socrates' line, "The only true wisdom is knowing you know nothing." To me that signifies that you should always keep your mind open in anticipation of more learning. Sounds like good advice for lifelong learning.

Having been drawn to study Positive Psychology during the writing of this book, it seems fitting and appropriate that I include a discussion of the five character strengths of wisdom as they are presented in *Character Strengths and Virtues: A Handbook and Classification.*[18]

In *Character Strengths and Virtues*, the authors identify six universal virtues: Wisdom and Knowledge, Courage, Humanity, Justice, Temperance, and Transcendence. They define wisdom as "knowledge hard fought for, and then used for good." The character strengths of wisdom include the following:

- Creativity
- Curiosity
- Open-Mindedness
- Love of Learning
- Perspective (Wisdom)[19]

Isn't it interesting that all five of the character strengths are topics included in this book?

Following are examples of how the character strengths can be used:[20]

- **Creativity**: thinking up a new story to tell your child
- **Curiosity**: asking a neighbor a couple of questions
- **Open-Mindedness**: reading two very different news columns to get different views
- **Love of Learning**: reading three online articles about the same topic
- **Perspective**: offering a one-liner of advice to a clerk who seems to be having a bad day

To learn more about your strengths, there is a link to the VIA Character Strengths Survey in the Resources section at the end of this book.

While most psychologists agree that wisdom involves an integration of knowledge, experience, and deep understanding, it also incorporates listening with your heart and being open and receptive when listening to other people and when responding to them.

Scientists disagree whether wisdom increases with age or not. Some studies have found that it does, while others have not. However, I tend to believe it does. What is my empirical evidence? Over fifty interviews with Inclined Elders from 40 to 100 who continue to climb the hill and live life with meaning and purpose. These older people have not bought into society's negative connotation of aging as a time of inevitable decline and being over-the-hill. They are all marching to the beat of their own drums—continuing to climb the hill and Incline—with meaning and purpose. That to me demonstrates wisdom.

Can wisdom be measured? Only in the last decade has this been possible due largely to the work of Professor Monika Ardelt. She developed a wisdom scoring model that can be used to find out your own wisdom score.[21]

Professor Ardelt provides suggestions on becoming wise:

- **Observe Everything**: open your eyes and really see all that is in your surroundings
- **Be Mindful**: practice "mindful presence" and "mindful listening" when speaking with someone
- **Move Towards Meditation**: practice spending time with yourself, rather than just by yourself[22]

I like Socrates' words of advice in Plato's Republic: "I enjoy talking with very old people. They have gone before us on a road by which we, too, may have to travel, and I think we do well to learn from them what it is like." I'd say that back in the day, Socrates knew a lot of Incliners and no doubt was one himself.

You may recall at the end of the Introduction I asked you to ponder the following:

> *The 18th century English poet William Wordsworth once wrote: "The wiser mind mourns less for what age takes away than what it leaves behind." As you read this book, think about what you would most like to jettison, in order to feel lighter and free, as you learn how best to live YOUR life of Incline.*

I made the same suggestion to Herb (The Eternal Incliner), age 100, and Lee (Keep the Inner Child Alive), age 95.

Herb: The Eternal Incliner—Wisdom

Herb was born in Germany in 1919. As the Nazi party gained power in the 1930s, Herb's family was persecuted. They managed to obtain a visa for him, and he was sent to live with a cousin in the United States. Herb completed his university undergraduate degree and became a naturalized US citizen. He enlisted in the US Army and served three and one-half years in combat in Europe during World War II.

> At a recent dinner with the co-president of our retirement community, one resident called me "An Old

Historical Guy." We all got a good laugh about it. But then I could look back to an almost 100-year life so filled with sadness, filled with depression, and yes mourning, fears, and feelings of inadequacies. However, also a life of accomplishments, joyfulness, pride, and satisfaction.

As I near the 100-year marker, I am daily aware of the loss of independence. As in my earlier life, I have adjusted to it. Physically, I feel the difficulties, occasionally pain in getting around, having caregivers entering my daily life routine. Yet I have a need to stay active, creative, whether it's financial work, staying in touch with friends, all younger generations than my own. Reading books, magazines, newspapers, watching news programs on TV, being part of a writing group, public speaking, taking weekly yoga and fitness classes.

What gives me more satisfaction in this long life is being the patriarch of a large, accomplished, and devoted family. Although we are scattered geographically, we stay in close touch and we celebrate our togetherness pretty regularly. Last but by no means least, I have been married almost seventy-three years, yes, to the same woman. Cathy has shared my life throughout this long and exciting journey.

I have no regrets. If anything, I often marvel at all the events I was a part of. Staying alive during three and one-half years of combat, being reviewed by Franklin Roosevelt and Winston Churchill. Being introduced to General de Gaulle. Being part of the great crusade—D-Day June 6, 1944. Being awarded the Legion of Honor by the French government. These are but a few that have come to mind in a long, eventful life. I guess I am "A Historical Guy" with lots of luck on my side. Oh, and I can say with much pride I am a member of the Greatest Generation. And when taps is blown on Memorial Day, I weep for all the comrades I have lost on this journey—all those who were a part of my life.

For Herb, many years filled with sadness, depression, mourning and fears are far outweighed by a life of accomplishments, joyfulness, pride, and satisfaction.

Lee: Keep the Inner Child Alive—Wisdom

Lee was born in Palestine, Texas, in 1924. She is an amazing woman who has overcome many life challenges. At fifty Lee began a successful career as an inspiring motivational speaker and is now the oldest living member of the National Speakers Association. In 2013 she was awarded the Lifetime Achievement Award by the National Speakers Association Austin Chapter. Her inner child is alive and kicking in her ninety-fifth year.

I could certainly write a chapter about all my forty-one surgeries, a horrible divorce, being rejected by my only son for thirty-one years, almost total conflict with my mother for seventy years, losing a large percentage of my hearing and the ability to walk freely, fighting cancer twice (eleven surgeries), and the latest—recently having to surrender my driver's license! No way to escape it, but we can do a lot to help ourselves in managing it. You know it is up to each of us to prepare for it as best we can! Attitude is everything!

What I think about Wordsworth's statement is: I partially agree with him. I have come to realize that old age can be a series of losing people and things most dear to us. It can be a horrible trap for those who suffer from physical or mental ailments that cannot be healed, leaving a huge, empty hole. And a multitude of negative things can happen to us about which we have no control. Losing a loved one can be devastating! It is true: "Old age is not for sissies!" I have come to realize that the only thing we do have control over is how we think! Therefore, older people who have learned to keep their sense of humor, to think positively, who genuinely care for other people and REMAIN ACTIVE, who continue to learn and are still interested in life in general, who do not let their INNER CHILD fade away, definitely can "mourn less for what age takes away then what it leaves behind"!

Lee's last sentence sums it up nicely. And don't forget the "attitude" that she mentioned earlier on.

My call to action for you is to use your wisdom as Incliners to challenge the existing social reality. Aging is NOT all about decline. Demonstrate to society that as Inclined Elders we're still climbing the hill and loving it!

PERSONAL REFLECTIONS

1. How can you contribute to a societal change in perception—from one of decline to one of continuing Incline?
   Consider the ways included in chapter 5 in the Culture section.

2. To what degree do you possess knowledge and wisdom?
   Consider knowledge and wisdom on a continuum. If knowledge is having an understanding of certain information and wisdom is the ability to use your knowledge to make good decisions, where do you fall on the continuum?

PART 3

EMPOWERMENT

*"You cannot control what happens to you,
but you can control your attitude toward what
happens to you, and in that, you will be mastering
change rather than allowing it to master you."*

~ Sri Ram, a major deity of Hinduism

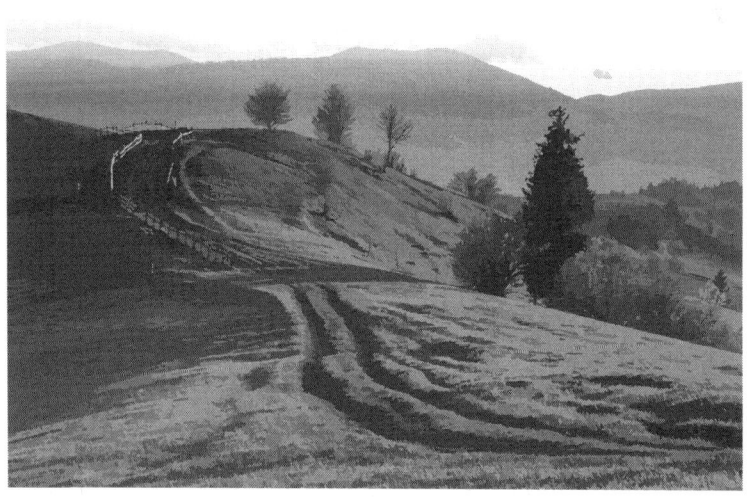

CHAPTER 6

LEAVE A LEGACY AND LIVE IT NOW

Whether you think you can,
or you think you can't—you're right."
~ **Henry Ford**

Empowerment is the process of becoming stronger and more confident, especially in gaining control over your own life. "It is a process that fosters power in people for use in their own lives, their communities, and in their society by acting on issues that they define as important."[1]

As you've travelled on this journey with the Inclined Elders, you've become more aware that you have the free will to:

- Adopt a positive attitude with respect to aging
- Choose to commit to a meaningful, purposeful life of Incline as you get older

- Make every day count
- Add movement to your life
- Strive for continuous growth through:
  - Social engagement—relationships and community
  - Life course model of life
  - Lifelong learning
- Understand cultural differences
- Embrace your personal wisdom

You have been moving towards embracing your own power. You are becoming stronger, more confident. You are now ready to take control—of your own life. If you choose to do so.

The following stories demonstrate how some Inclined Elders embraced their power.

Dora: Migrant to MBA

Imagine a beautiful little five-year old girl sitting by the edge of a field gazing at her parents. They are migrant farmworkers, and she is waiting for them to come in from a long day of toil. She loves her parents dearly, but they are laborers working labor type jobs, and she determines she doesn't want to do this. She doesn't want that kind of life. What thoughts do you think are swirling in her head?

As Dora recalls, "I knew even when I was five years old that an education was going to change that. But I also knew that my family didn't understand." They obviously wanted the best for her, and when she was in high school and told her parents she was going to go to college, they said okay. But it was like when a child comes home and says they're going to be a singer or an actress and the parents say, "Okay, dear." Those are things that other people do. This is not what Dora's family did.

Getting a higher education and going into the workforce was just not something Dora grew up with. That wasn't something that was expected of her. It wasn't even something that was supported in the beginning because it wasn't understood in her Hispanic culture. So it was quite a surprise to everyone when she announced she wanted to go to university after high school. Everyone wondered how and why she was going to do that. What was she going to do? Why wasn't she getting married and having children like the rest of them?

But Dora knew her mind. She persevered with resolve and many years later earned both a bachelor's and a master's degree. She is the first person in her family to do so.

The biggest thing for Dora, and she still questions this a lot, was her identity. She had to leave all the things that she had been growing up and be somebody else to be successful academically and in her professional career. But she felt it was okay and believed you don't have to give up your dreams, who you want to be.

Today, Dora's family is very proud of her accomplishments. By embracing self-empowerment and fulfilling her dream, Dora provided inspiration for her children. They've never questioned that they will get a college degree. She has bestowed that sense of empowerment to her children. The seeds have been planted.

As we explored in the previous chapter, a social or cultural norm is the behavioral expectation that a social group holds for its individuals.[2] Dora was able to break free from the expectation of her culture that she would get married, have children, and be a homemaker, as her family and ancestors had done before her. She was able to follow her dream.

She continued her education at university, earned two degrees, and today enjoys a successful career in academia. But most importantly, she has left a legacy of empowerment for her children and future generations.

Polly: Introversion to Volunteerism

After teaching kindergarten and elementary children for over thirty years, Polly decided to retire when she learned she was going to be a grandmother. She offered to take care of Paulina, the joy of her life, while her mom and dad ran their café. This was Polly's focus for five years until her granddaughter started kindergarten. When that day arrived, she was left with a lot of time on her hands. What was she going to do with it? Polly shared, "I really had to push myself to get out of the house to try new things because I am extremely introverted. It was hard for me at first. But I wanted to find something I could do that gave me that sense of reward I got from teaching."

In order to accomplish this, Polly started looking for volunteer opportunities in her neighborhood. She wanted to do something political that helped people get involved. She located an ad for volunteers to assist people with disabilities to vote. She thought she'd love to help because she'd been a special education teacher working with disabled students for years. This was something she could do.

Even though she considers herself an introvert, Polly mustered her courage to attend the meeting. She remembers, "I was really nervous because I was going somewhere I'd never been before and I would be around people I'd never met. But when the organizer reached out her hand to greet me, she said I was going to meet some amazing people. She worded it in a way that was so inviting. I thought I could do this and I'm so glad I did." As she shared this story with me, her face glowed with pride.

Polly further recalls, "I really did have to push myself because the more you stay at home and the more you are kind of isolated, the harder it is to get out. It was hard for me because I'm introverted, and I can be very shy. But I'm so glad I did push myself because I feel more confident. I feel more courageous and I now think, well if I did that, then I can do something else. I now go to places I've never been to before. I walk in and meet people and talk to people I don't know. And I ask people if they'd like to register to vote. All of this has really been fun."

A sense of helping people has expanded Polly's horizons. "I'm feeling good about what I'm doing so it helps me as much as it helps the people I'm working with. It really is important to me to give back and do something that is meaningful."

Today, at sixty-five, Polly has expanded her volunteer work and is now teaching pre-reading and early reading skills at Paulina's school.

While admittedly still an introvert, Polly was able to overcome her initial shyness of exploring new opportunities to regain that sense of reward she got from teaching.

The concepts of introversion and extroversion were introduced in 1921 by Carl Jung, a Swiss psychoanalyst. Jung saw these two concepts on a continuum with extreme introversion at one end and extreme extroversion at the other. While we all have characteristics of both, generally, one of these inborn traits is more dominant than the other.[3]

Jung believed that the difference between the two is all about energy. While extroverts direct their energy outwards—towards other people—and gain energy from these encounters, introverts focus their energy inwards, towards more solitary, thoughtful activities. People that tend to fall somewhere in between on the introversion-extroversion continuum are considered "ambivert," and they display characteristics of both.[4]

Introversion can look like shyness, but that is not necessarily the case. An introvert enjoys time alone and their energy level may dip after spending time with a lot of people. A shy person may not want to be alone but may be reluctant to interact with others. Not all introverts are shy. If introversion is your dominant character trait, this will remain with you during your lifetime. However, shyness can be overcome through personal work, such as Polly's determination to attend that first meeting, or counseling.[5]

Polly was able to successfully overcome her initial feeling of shyness by mustering her courage and taking that first step to attend the volunteer meeting.

If you experience a sense of discomfort in making a change in your life and trying something different, take a lesson from Polly. Start a new activity or project. In so doing, you may gain a sense of reward like Polly found from volunteering.

If you want to increase your confidence, the article entitled "4 Ways to Increase Your Confidence from the Inside Out"[6] might be helpful. A link is available in the Resources section at the end of this book.

You often hear that we cannot love and care for others if we don't love and care for ourselves first. Self-love, self-care, and self-compassion are important themes when considering empowerment.[7]

Suzanne: Recipe for Love

"Knowing my family and friends love me makes me feel confident, a stronger woman, and more empowered. I feel deeply honored to experience this loving feeling inside because I am who I am: a daughter, sister, wife, mother, grandmother, friend."

At sixty-nine, Suzanne views love from several perspectives. She believes it's important to share the little things we love with family and friends. Suzanne shared, "I love items such as shoes, heart-shaped objects, boxes, to name a few. This is part of me and makes me who I am. Ben, one of my grandsons, and I share a love of olives. He often buys me olives as gifts, and I always have a special dish of olives at his place setting when he comes to dinner. When my family and friends acknowledge my favorite things, they let me know they are thinking of me, and I know they love me. I, in turn, can express my love back to them with gifts of little things they love."

Another aspect of love for Suzanne is food. For her, having special dinners for family and friends is one of the best ways to express your love. They know you've gone the extra mile when you serve a special dish and spend valuable time with them.

A love of nature is central to Suzanne's core essence. She expressed, "I feel very spiritual when I am hiking in the forest. My entire being feels calm and peaceful. I thank God I'm alive and for the wonderful people I have in my life that I love." Fishing with her husband, Raymond, is one of her favorite things to do with him. Suzanne said, "When we're in the boat together, we make our five-year plans, talk about other topics, or just sit quietly and look at each other, thankful we are together."

How we look at life is always a choice. Do we want to view it with fear and anger, and struggle against it? Or do we want to allow it, accept it, and eventually embrace it?[8] Why not love ourselves just the way we are? Life's journey is about universal love. It's about learning to love. Love yourself and you can then love others, as they can love you. This paves the way to freedom.

I invite you to develop a loving relationship with your age and aging. As shared in a previous chapter, I'm "just" seventy and I'm proud of it. Don't fight it! Embrace it!

Jonathan: Self Love Revolution

After beating himself up for years, Jonathan came to the realization that he didn't love himself very much. It was at this turning point he began to develop his Self Love Revolution program based on his training, readings, and personal studying.

Many of Jonathan's clients come to him with a sense of self-loathing, a sense of self-doubt that they are not able to accomplish something in their lives that they are seeking. Jonathan believes that we all wear different masks for different people. We're never really showing up as ourselves. And the person we're talking to has their own mask on. So, as Jonathan explains, "What we have is a mask talking to a mask. We have no idea who the other person is or what they really think. So, self-love is an opportunity to show up as who you are and to give others permission to show up as who they are. And just perhaps two people can talk to each other as real people not as the masks that we think the other person wants to see."

The mission of the Self Love Revolution is to help people find the joy inside of them. How is this done? Jonathan states, "We're all born with joy. But as we age somehow that sense of joy can become buried within us. But it's always there. If you feel you've lost it, just peel back the layers. Because you're either growing or you're dying. And you get to choose whether you want today to be a day of growth or a day of dying." Jonathan's Self Love Revolution program accomplishes this.

How does the Self Love Revolution work? What is the methodology for finding the joy inside yourself again?

The methodology consists of Four Pillars:

- **Acceptance:** complete acceptance of what is and of the fact that you may want it to be different. When you accept both, you stop fighting with yourself, your body, your brain, the stories. You just stop fighting. That's what acceptance is. It stops fighting. And once you stop fighting you can add the next pillar.
- **Gratitude:** a rewiring of the brain to look for joyous things in the world. Focusing on the positive things. And it's hormonal too. Expressing gratitude releases serotonin, which stabilizes the body.
- **Forgiveness:** forgiving yourself, not just others
- **Kindness:** being kind to yourself daily

The Four Pillars of Jonathan's Self Love Revolution methodology lend themselves perfectly to living a life of Incline.

Self-love is a practice just like brushing your teeth. You need to do it every day. It's simply a new habit we need to form.

At fifty-three Jonathan believes that if we can get a few people to begin to practice self-love—and hopefully thousands or millions of people begin to practice and share it with others—then we'll have a better world. He shared, "When people love themselves, they are not so quick to hate other people. It all has to do with the fear of ourselves. When we love ourselves, we don't see the differences so much between ourselves and others. There is simply more unity. That's the legacy."

Aligned with Jonathan's self-love program is the construct of self-compassion. Instead of judging and criticizing yourself for various shortcomings, when practicing self-compassion you are kind and understanding when confronted with your personal failings.[9]

Dr. Kristin Neff, one of the leading experts on self-compassion, contends there are three elements of self-compassion:

1. **Self-kindness vs. Self-judgment:** being warm and understanding towards yourself
2. **Common humanity vs. Isolation:** recognizing that personal inadequacy is part of shared human experience

3. **Mindfulness over Over-identification:** taking a balanced approach to our negative emotions[10]

Find out how self-compassionate you are. Take the test in the Resources section at the end of this book.

Edith: Kids Life Mastery

Edith's husband Jonathan shared, "With Edith's Kids Life Mastery program, she really is teaching self-love for the future. She's changing the way it's taught to children. She's changing it on a societal level. Then these kids learn they can Incline their whole lives."

The mission of Kids Life Mastery is "transforming kids' lives, not just today, but every day in the future." It's a research-based coaching program designed by Edith to help kids master their own lives in the midst of the chaotic world we live in. Students learn how to live their own lives, on their own terms, and how to guarantee their own success as they define it. At forty-one this is the work that Edith is passionate about.

When Edith and Jonathan moved from Los Angeles to Austin, Edith left a successful career in healthcare, where she had done clinical work with veterans and their families and social work with kids and families. They had just had their son, Mateo. As a new mom with no career, it hit Edith hard that she had to redefine herself. She reflected, "I was no longer the person I'd been in LA. I was now Jonathan's wife. I was Mateo's mom. But who was I?"

That's how Kids Life Mastery was born. It was a culmination of everything in Edith's life. Her growth and her failings. She felt like there was so much to share that it was important to give that back to the kids. Edith shared, "So the idea came to me. Why couldn't I apply the research on failing and success I'd applied to myself to the younger generation? Just having vulnerable, open, honest conversations with younger generations about what's to come or what to look forward to is important. It's a part of the work that I do every single day. And that to me is my responsibility and how I can give back."

Edith started working with tweens and teens and now works with children as young as five years old. As she related, "It's awesome. Kids are so receptive, so incredibly smart, and in tune with life. When I wrote the program, it was for tweens and teens and I thought no, truly this cannot work with five-year-olds, but sure enough it does." So, what is the program? It's teaching kids to master their own lives and empowering them to make their own life decisions, independent of the beliefs of their parents or society or school.

Now four years into the program, Edith has worked with over 200 kids at the studio and in schools. The ones that always come to mind are the kids that have social anxiety. She teaches them to go inside of their bodies—to just be aware of what's going on—and experience gratitude and acceptance. A child's transformation is a gift to them, and witnessing and being a part of it is a gift to her.

~

As discussed in chapter 5, ageism abounds in our society through the practice of stereotyping older adults. By acknowledging and embracing your age, you can take the first step on the path of self-empowered aging, thereby positioning yourself to make your later years as productive and purposeful as possible.[11]

Self-empowered aging is taking control of your life, continuing to learn, taking risks, making changes, and developing the resilience to overcome challenges. There are many roads to self-empowerment, including:

- Return to school or lifelong learning
- Continue to work
- Pursue an encore career
- Start a business[12]

The options are endless. Embrace with gratitude the experience of aging and the challenge of taking on ageism through self-empowerment."[13]

ROLE MODELS

At the beginning of the book I posited that because we're living longer, we have an important choice to make: Commit to a meaningful, purposeful life of Incline as we get older, or believe that a new stage—one of steady decline—is inevitable.

Invariably the men and women whose personal journeys you've just experienced made the choice to commit to a meaningful, purposeful life of Incline. They opted not to accept society's negative connotation that aging is a new stage of steady decline.

Numerous surveys have been conducted that indicate younger adults have a negative attitude towards aging, no doubt based on society's negative connotation and all the media hype. One such report, "That Age Old Question," polled a group of twenty- and thirty-year-olds. Overall, they were found to have the most negative attitudes about aging and older people, compared to other age groups. Some of the results included:

- 40% believe that there isn't any way to escape dementia as you age
- 25% believe it's normal to be unhappy and depressed when you are old
- 24% think older people can never really be thought of as attractive
- 64% don't have a single friendship with an age gap of thirty years or more[14]

No wonder many young people do not look forward to the prospect of aging.

My premise is that if young adults have positive older role models in their lives, Incliners who are continuing to climb the hill, they will be more receptive to aging. To test my theory, I interviewed several younger adults in their twenties and thirties to determine their attitude towards aging. I asked them what old means to them? Did they have an older role model and, if so, was there a positive impact? And what was their attitude towards growing older?

Is it possible to dispel our society's myth of aging as inevitable decline and younger adults' negative attitude towards aging? The young adults featured below are just some examples of the broader understanding that can help us, collectively, shift away from our current society's derision of "old age." As you read their perspectives, consider how important personal influencers have been in helping these young people regard aging in a more positive way. Hopefully, this will help you understand the importance of becoming one of those influencers yourself.

Briana: Behavior Matters

Briana is an artist and she applies her creativity to all aspects of her professional and personal life. At twenty-six, Briana's entrepreneurial spirit drives her career—from writing for social impact organizations to marketing and advertising for tech companies. She loves it all.

"I think 'old' has to do with behavior. When someone is close-minded to new experiences, opportunities, and learning, it ages them. When older people are set in their ways, to me that feels like a product of being old. So open-mindedness and behavior are critical. I know some adults who act older than ninety-eight-year-old Betty White and ninety-four-year-old Dick Van Dyke. Both are definitely young at heart."

Who was a role model for Briana and what made the connection? "I've always been a learner and high on everything to do with it—high input, high learner, high achiever—so I think trying to connect with people in my life that can be in a mentorship role is personally appealing. I love the idea of them handing off some of that wisdom or coaching to me. Growing up, my best friend was my grandma and she was my mentor for many years."

Briana is excited about growing older. She's addicted to the idea that there's opportunity in everything one does, every new experience. So, there's potential for enormous growth. She looks forward to her thirties, forties, and beyond, but Briana doesn't want to rush it. She wants to savor every year.

Briana likes to joke with people whenever they mention, "Oh my God, this year's flown by." Why?

"When you think about it, it makes sense because every year is like an exponentially shrinking slice of the pie. It's relatively shorter. Like every year I'm living now is $1/26^{th}$ of my life. When you're four it's $1/4^{th}$ of your life. When you're eighty that's $1/80^{th}$ of your life. When you're down to the second, each second seems relatively shorter than the last second. That freaks people out but I think it's fascinating. That means I'll be less reactive, less defensive, I'll care less. That means I won't take things so personally. Every year that you mature maybe you'll be less jaded or maybe you'll see things from different perspectives. Whatever you decide. It's your choice. And that's exciting.

"With regard to wisdom, I feel when people live more life they have more to share. But I think a large percentage of it just comes from their perspective and the more point of view you gain the more perspective you are exposed to as you get older because you just naturally meet more people or interact with more people. I think that just allows you to have greater wisdom and understanding."

Briana's perspective is illuminating. What wisdom at such a young age to be so positive that every year she ages she'll be less jaded and "I'll care less" because she realizes it's her choice.

Hailey: Texting with PawPaw

Hailey is a rising star with a Manhattan tech company. At twenty-three, she considers "old" a flexible term and not a number. She views it as being more mature, being more knowledgeable, or having more experience than she does.

Her oldest friend was her grandfather, PawPaw. They would talk or text daily as she walked from her apartment to the subway on her way to work. She reached out to him often, asking him for advice. "He had such an amazingly cool life. He had a unique outlook. If I questioned something or wanted an opinion, he always gave me straight advice, no baloney. I valued his wisdom. Something he always told me was to 'watch my six,' which translates to watch your back. He told me this was a phrase they used during his time in the military. So, every phone call ended with love you and watch your six."

Hailey continued, "I've been blessed to know my grandparents and they have changed my outlook towards elders. Because of them, I'm excited to get older."

What a special relationship between a grandfather and granddaughter with an over sixty-year age difference. Testament to the power of older role models in young peoples' lives.

Jody: The Same Playing Field

At thirty-six, Jody understands the importance of positive role models in our lives. Nancy J was Jody's first real boss after she earned her master's in college and entered the workforce. She has been a tremendous influence in her life. Nancy taught her to embrace life and be present in every moment. She also pushed planning for the future. Nancy served as her greatest mentor.

When asked what the value is of having older friends, Jody responded, "Definitely a sense of wisdom and an emphasis that we all have choices in our lives." Jody isn't stuck on a number when she thinks of old age. "It's more about quality of life. If I'm living life, doing things that bring me joy, that's a good quality of life." What does Jody consider as advantages to growing older? "Wisdom, freedom to have new adventures, mindset, definitely gratitude. Instead of dreading it, I'm excited."

One of the most important lessons Nancy taught Jody concerns mindset. The thing that differentiates people with degrees of success and happiness is their mindset. In a nutshell everybody comes from different backgrounds. You might have grown up rich. You might have grown up poor. You might have grown up educated or uneducated. As Jody asserts, "But at the end of the day, every single person has the same number of hours in each day. What you do with those hours positively or negatively frames your entire life. We're all on the same playing field when it comes to what we do with our life. Your mindset makes the most difference in your entire life."

Another excellent example of how we all can choose how to live our lives.

Chris and Ashley: Shuffleboard on the Ice

At forty and thirty-four, Chris and Ashley lead a very active life. In addition to enjoying their horses and other animals, they are members of a local curling team.

Chris and Ashley introduced me to three senior athletes in the sport of curling. On their team the skip, also known as the captain, is Brian. He is a retired truck driver with well over forty years of curling experience. He has competed all over Canada, including the highest level in Canadian curling, the Labatt Brier. In third position, as the vice skip, is Donna. She is an administrator for an active oilfield company. Donna has been playing in the sport for over twenty-five years. In second position is Roy. He is a retired dairy farmer who not only participates in the sport but creates and maintains the ice surface at the local arena.

Next is Chris and Ashley's position on the team, lead. They are the first to throw the stones. As the youngest, they take turns sharing this position and strive to curl at the level of the more senior members.

Chris and Ashley shared, "These three friends and team-mates have an average age of sixty. From them we gain both curling and life skills—on and off the ice. Our diverse ages within the team has not hindered us. Rather it has been a benefit when enjoying the sport of curling."

Steve: Cross-Country Ski Challenge

About twelve years ago Steve and his wife, Bobbi-Jo, went on a cross-country ski trip. It was a clear but very cold day at -20C (approximately -4F). They made good time and arrived at a warming cabin about halfway through the journey. Steve got a fire going to warm the little shelter. Through the window he spotted a couple slowly skiing towards the cabin. When he opened the door, he was amazed.

As he shared, "There was an older man in his late eighties or early nineties and his wife of the same vintage. He wore wool everywhere with knee-high wool gaiters, and he had a small day pack. He was happy to get inside the cabin and was impressed that we had got a fire going. He said, 'You never know what you get in the cabin for dry wood, so I bring my own.' He then opened his pack and took out precut cedar kindling and homemade fire starters and stoked the fire. We kept talking and learned that he is a regular cross-country skier and a little cold doesn't bother him."

Steve was so impressed that this older man and his wife could continue to be active and enjoy themselves. It confirmed for him that getting old doesn't mean quitting the things that you love to do.

At thirty-seven, Steve has not spent a lot of time thinking about aging. He knows it will come but he's in no way prepared for it. "I do try to eat right and exercise but that has a benefit right now as well. I am not afraid to age and get older, and I know that it is all part of life."

Steve hopes to age slowly and continue to do the things that he loves to do with his family and friends. As he said, "I would be very pleased if I could cross-country ski in my nineties, packing my own wood and GORP" (GORP = Good Old Raisins and Peanuts).

Bobbi-Jo: Nursing and Bagpipes

While nursing in acute medicine, Bobbi-Jo had a great deal of exposure to an aging population. In the early years of nursing, she often thought to herself, "Ugh, I don't want to 'get old'!" Bobbi-Jo worked with patients and families who were experiencing chronic and acute conditions or changes to their health. There were many challenging times caring for people who were in pain, experiencing various degrees of loss (physical, mental), and dying. However, there was also inspiration seeing people recover and leave the hospital to return home to their lives.

Bobbi-Jo loved it when ladies in the hospital would do their hair, get dressed, and put on their lipstick. Although not at home, they still got up and ready for the day ahead. She will always remember one patient who was 102 years old and was using a smart phone to chat with her family.

"It took a while, but at some point, I started to realize that the tiny population of people being cared for in a hospital is not a reflection of all the older people living in our community. I started to think more positively about all the people not in the hospital."

On another note, Bobbi-Jo shared her involvement with her Pipe and Drum Band. The band has a few younger members, but it's made up mostly of men and women who are over age sixty-five. In fact, one member learned to play the bagpipes at age seventy. The band was founded thirty-five years ago. The gentleman who started the band has just retired at age eighty. Through the decades, he has been a committed leader, teacher, and mentor.

"It's inspiring to see older people getting out, playing music, marching in parades (in all kinds of weather), learning new tunes, and competing in band competitions and events. To top it off, they always have a good joke and great stories to tell! These aren't the kind of people who sit around complaining about their age or ailments, nor do I overhear conversations about regret. I view these people as my friends and respect their passion for music and community."

Bobbi-Jo concluded, "I used to dread the thought of aging, but these days I am mindful of the positive things in life and, at thirty-seven, I look forward to the experiences that come with living—at any age."

Three Generations of Incliners

I'm convinced that Inclining runs in a family. Herb (The Eternal Incliner), introduced at the beginning of the book and featured in the wisdom section, is an amazing gentleman. And at 100 he's still Inclining.

He obviously passed that philosophy on to his daughter, Nancy SB (The Eternal Dancer), and in turn to his grandsons, Ian, age thirty-two, and Colin, twenty-eight. I asked Ian and Colin to share their thoughts regarding the positive impact their grandfather has made on their perception of aging. They provided the following. Proof indeed that, because of the positive role models of their parents and grandparents, they are optimistic about aging and getter older.

Ian

•

"What I find the most striking about Grandpa Herb is his consistently positive and jovial attitude. He reminds me to laugh and not let anything get in the way of enjoying myself. I feel that many people lose this part of their personality as they age and have to face loss and other hardships, but it is important to remind yourself not to take life too seriously or it will not be enjoyable to live to such an old age."

Colin

"My grandfather's longevity and his nearly infallible memory gave me the perception that most people in the eighth and ninth decades of their life acted the way he does. His sense of humor and personality have stayed with him consistently, aspects which I do not think could ever be lost for him. He has also maintained an independent and active lifestyle until his mid-nineties. His life brings into perspective how much the world has changed within one hundred years, while his memories can be recalled as if they happened yesterday. My grandfather makes me hopeful about getting older. He demonstrates how insignificant age is compared to one's perceptions of life."

Four Generations of Incliners

I'm proud to share that four generations of my Inclining family are included in this book. Remember my mother who kicked up her heels and did a little dance just for the sheer joy of it when she was happy? Vera was an Incliner and innately knew it. I and my brother, Raymond, and sister-in-law, Suzanne, have followed in that tradition and are still Inclining. Chris and Ashley and Steve and Bobbi-Jo as young adults have been positively influenced by older role models in their lives. No doubt Ben and Matty, Steve and Bobbi-Jo's sons, at eight and six, have an attitude of Inclining embedded in their genes.

I highly recommend having friends of many ages, young and old. What a gift for you and them to share your lives with each other. It truly will be enriching.

LEGACY

"Legacy is not leaving something for people.
It's leaving something in people."

~ **Peter Strople**

Why Legacy?

Every day we are confronted with choices. What are some of yours? To:

- Determine a life of continuing Incline or accept that it's mostly downhill from here?
- Welcome change or feel more comfortable with the status quo?

• Embrace your authenticity or prefer not to make waves at this point?

These are important questions because the totality of our choices becomes our life and, in turn, determines the kind of legacy we leave.

Legacy is generally defined as a gift or bequest that is handed down from one person to another. However, true legacy can also be the quality of your life overall. But, beyond that, think of the choices you make and the actions you take as having a ripple effect that can positively (or not!) impact your family, your friends, your communities, and society. Certainly, it's motivating to know that when you shift to living with a mindset of legacy, you are choosing a more authentic life path for yourself.

But isn't it even more inspiring to realize that you have the means—in every moment of every day—with which to encourage the next—or even later—generations to aspire and work towards realizing their own potential?

Creating a true legacy is a pathway that leads to a deeper sense of empowerment well beyond the pursuit of wealth or success.

Older adults can serve as role models and leave a legacy of Incline for future generations. And what better generation than the Boomers to demonstrate this momentum, being the first generation with an extended life span and a desire for "changing aging."

We can become an inspiring example so our society relinquishes the notion that aging is synonymous with "decline," "decrepit," "senile," and "over-the-hill" once and for all. Rather than settling for a life of complacency, conventionality, and compliance, we choose to embrace change, curiosity, and courage.

That's certainly a credo to live by and one I attest to. While reinventing myself several times over—both personally and professionally—I have always remained true to my core essence. I release those things that no longer serve me. I choose to live my legacy now by serving as a role model for future generations and society. Because one of the strongest ways we can make changes is by modeling the behaviors and values we believe in and helping others on that path. How about you?

Quality of Life or Quantity of Years?

Which do you consider more important: quality of life or quantity of years? Historically, or so it seems, the emphasis has been mostly one way, quantity of years. I intend—with your help—to change that.

Since time immemorial, there always have been those who have sought to prolong life. Take Gilgamesh, a 2000 BCE king in an epic, who sought a longevity-granting plan. In the sixteenth century Ponce de Leon was a Spanish explorer who ventured to new lands supposedly seeking the fountain of youth. In Oscar Wilde's *The Picture of Dorian*

Gray, the hero sold his soul for eternal youth. All sought eternal life and all failed.

Fast-forward to today and there are still those who continue the quest for either increased longevity or eternal youth. A group of successful Silicon Valley entrepreneurs have been trying for years to reconfigure death.[15]

And yet there are people that are of the opinion that they'd rather opt for quality of life and just as soon have their life end as they reach their peak. Their opinion is that society and families—and you—would be better off if nature takes its course swiftly and promptly.[16]

Would you like to live to 100 years or beyond? The probability of living to at least 100 for those born today is 50%.[17]

While this is all well and good, there is an alternative path to consider as we age. Let's combine quantity with quality. I suggest you choose an attitude of Incline so that you're continuing to climb hills and living your best life irrespective of how old you are.

What Society Needs to Do

Sociologists study how individuals behave in groups and how their behavior is shaped by these groups or life models.[18] At this time in our evolution we need to reevaluate our existing life model based on the facts:

- The existing one no longer works, as it evolved for lives that were half as long.

- Our traditional three-stages of life—education, work and family, retirement—is outdated.
- A new life course is required to provide greater flexibility and multiple stages.[19]

A new model is needed that will support people to live high-quality lives for 100 years or more, including:

- New models for education, including lifelong learning
- A redesign of how we work
- New policies for healthcare, housing, the environment
- More intergenerational communities[20]

Many groups of forward-thinking individuals are studying ways to do this. One such group is the Stanford Center on Longevity. The center launched a five-year initiative in 2018 that focuses on deep dives into the above areas. The goal is to begin to lay groundwork for cultures that support century-long lives.[21] The aim is to develop recommendations for governments, employers, businesses, parents, and policymakers. This initiative is called a "New Map of Life."

Laura Carstensen is a professor of psychology and director of the Stanford Center on Longevity. She contends, "To make full use of longer lives, we need to radically change our thinking about how we live our lives from beginning to end."[22]

What You Need to Do

Yes, our society needs to change. But I believe change needs to start at a grassroots level. By this I mean each of us, including you. This is my "call to action" for you to look at your life and identity how you can become an Incliner. Following are some suggestions as featured in earlier chapters.

ATTITUDE

- **Make a Choice**
  Commit to a meaningful, purposeful life of Incline as you get older. (Introduction and Chapter 1)

- **Calamitous Cs vs Constructive Cs**
  Shed the shackles of the Calamitous Cs and embrace the Constructive Cs: Change, Curiosity, and Courage (Chapter 1)

- **Gratitude and Resilience**
  Begin practicing gratitude and your resilience level will increase. (Chapter 2)

- **Purpose and Planning**
  Identify a purpose in your life and make a plan to develop it. (Chapter 2)

- **Power of Play**
  Regain the inner child in you and rediscover the power of play. Get in touch with your sixth sense, proprioception, and get moving. As Amanda prescribes: movement is medicine. (Chapter 3)

GROWTH

- **Connections and Community**
  Increase the number of people in your life—of all ages. Choose a life course philosophy versus society's life stages. Embrace lifelong learning. (Chapter 5)

- **Culture and Wisdom**
  Understand that cultures are in transition. Use your growing wisdom as an Incliner to challenge the existing social perception of inevitable decline. (Chapter 5)

EMPOWERMENT

- **Self-Empowerment**
  As an Incliner you'll realize you are now embracing self-empowerment. You'll understand that by living your best life you are serving as a role model for future generations. In so doing, you are leaving a legacy and living it now.

You may think you're only one person, but if you share your newfound attitude of Inclining with others, you will be lighting a spark to ignite an explosion of new consciousness. As Margaret Mead, renowned cultural anthropologist, stated: "Never doubt that a small group of thoughtful, committed citizens can change the world; indeed, it's the only thing that ever has."

With Gratitude

I wish to express my gratitude to all the amazing Incliners that gave me the gift of their time and their stories. I am honored to be able to include them in *Inclined Elders*. Thank you all for your wisdom and for being here.

Return to the Beginning

I've enjoyed being your tour guide on this journey. Now it's time for you to begin the ascent and join us Incliners as we continue to climb the hill. As I pointed out at the beginning of this book, there's an amazing view from up here. Indeed, as we near the end of our journey, let's return to the beginning so we have come full circle. I'd like to leave you with part of my definition of Inclined Elders and once again invite you to join us.

The metaphor of a hill is an apt one to consider as you grapple with the concept of Inclining because hills are surely easier and more enjoyable to climb than steep, lofty mountains. And they still allow for inspiring discoveries and adventures. Some of their pathways may have twists and turns, and there may be the odd bump in the road, but it is important to continue the ascent. Why? Because the vistas on the trek upward are increasingly breathtaking and exhilarating.

Inclined Elders know that there's no need to rush; it's not a race. We take one step at a time, so we have the benefit of pausing to smile at the waving wildflowers along the road.

Your attitude determines the potential for your altitude, so a shift in mindset is required, regardless of your age right now. As you awaken to each new day as an Inclined Elder, the sunrise will greet you with a symphony of color applauding your choice to Incline and climb the hill. You will continue to broaden your experience and deepen your joy of life. It has for me and the people who shared their stories for this book.

Serving as vibrant role models, the Inclined Elders I spoke to for this book are leaving their own unique legacies of wisdom and inspiration for future generations. There needs to be more of us to effect real social change, so why not Incline too? There's an amazing view from up here. Come with us and see for yourself.

I look forward to seeing you on the path!

Ramona
Chief Incliner

PERSONAL REFLECTIONS

By choosing to live a life of Incline and continue to climb the hill, you will be embracing self-empowerment. You will be serving as a role model for future generations while living a meaningful and purposeful life now. What a legacy gift!

1. Are you currently living a life of Incline? If so, what positive impact has it had on your life?

2. Are you considering living a life of Incline? If so, what changes can you make in your current lifestyle to shift your mindset?

RESOURCES

I invite you to explore the many tips and techniques introduced below. Some of the resources are embedded in the chapters of the book, while others have been included only in this section. The purpose for gathering these resources is to provide you with supplemental material to that included in the book. They are additional tools or ideas to consider as you start living your life of Incline.

The Resources are grouped according to the specific benefit you can derive by reviewing them: Creativity, Gratitude, Positivity/Optimism, and Purpose. If the resource is embedded in the book, a reference will be provided below for the specific location. In the case of various tests that are available, a link has been included here. If a resource is from a book, a reference is listed.

I hope you enjoy these resources. I've tried them all. They are both interesting and thought-provoking.

The categories of resources are alphabetized as follow:

Creativity

1. It's Never Too Late to Begin Again

Gratitude

2. 3 Good Things
3. Angela's 3 Good Things Blog Article
4. Blessing and Gift Journal
5. Gratitude Quiz
6. Joy Buddy

Positivity/Optimism

7. 4 Ways to Increase Your Confidence from the Inside Out
8. Character Strengths and Virtues
9. Explanatory Style
10. Law of Attraction
11. Mindfulness
12. Positive Affirmations
13. Positivity Ratio
14. Self-Compassion Test
15. Thriving Quiz

Purpose

16. Ikigai
17. The Art of Contemplation

CREATIVITY

1. It's Never Too Late to Begin Again

While Julia Cameron's *The Artist's Way* provides a step-by-step process for people to recover and exercise their creativity, *It's Never Too Late* focuses on the older adult who is perhaps recently retired. By tapping into your internal creativity you will identify areas of interest and purpose in your life. Cameron's process provides principles for "creativity recovery."[1] This twelve-week course is for anyone transitioning into their second half of life, artist or otherwise. A few hours a week can become an amazing investment in the next phase of your life.

Basic Tools
Cameron provides a series of activities to aid in the "creativity recovery" process. They include:

- **Morning Pages:** three daily pages of longhand stream-of-consciousness writing done first thing in the morning
- **Memoirs:** a weekly process of triggering memories and revisiting your life
- **Artist Dates:** a weekly activity to explore something new and fun
- **Walking:** a twenty-minute solo walk twice a week[2]

So, buy a new journal, start exploring new locations for artist dates, and brush the dust off your walking shoes. Your creativity is about to be unleashed!

Expectation: Author's desire to answer "What next?" for students who are embarking on their 'second act.'"[3]
Location in Book: Chapter 3 (Creativity section)
Book Source: *It's Never Too Late to Begin Again,* Julia Cameron and Emma Lively

GRATITUDE

2. 3 Good Things

The link below is a video of Dr. Seligman presenting the 3 Good Things process.

Expectation: Increased gratitude, sense of well-being
Location in Book: Chapter 2 (Angela: 3 Good Things)
Book Source: *Authentic Happiness,* Martin Seligman
Website Link: https://www.youtube.com/ watch?v=ZOGAp9dw8Ac

3. Angela's 3 Good Things Blog Article

The link below will take you to Angela's 3 Good Things article.

Expectation: Increased gratitude, sense of well-being
Location in Book: Chapter 2 (Angela: 3 Good Things)
Website Link: https://www.linkedin.com/
pulse/3-good-things-angela-loeb

4. Blessing and Gift Journal

In her book, *Life's Companion*, Christina Baldwin outlines the process for keeping a blessing and gift journal as Carolyn has done for many years.

First off, treat yourself. Buy a new journal to use specifically for recording your blessings and gifts—perhaps a color that catches your eye. Or attach an image or saying on the cover that appeals to you. Use a pen that lends an easy flow to your writing.

A Blessing a Day
Before retiring each evening, pause and review your day. Write a brief comment, selecting one thing that was a gift from your day.

- It may be as simple as you heard the song of a bird early in the morning. It put a smile on your face and centered you for the rest of your day.

- While waiting in the checkout line at the market, you started chatting with the woman in front of you. You soon found you had lots in common. The brief chit-chat brightened your spirits.
- End each entry with "Thank you."[4]

A Gift a Day
In addition to daily receiving from the world, we also contribute. After noting your blessings for the day, pause and review your day again.

Write a brief statement about something that you gave back to the world today that you acknowledge as your gift.

- Perhaps you recognized an employee's good work on a project she's been working on for months. The broad smile that appeared on her face and her thank-you made you glow within.
- A friend is housebound due to an illness. You reached out to him by phone and offered your support in whatever way possible. He accepted. You'll be picking up and delivering a few groceries for him.
- End the entry with the words "You're welcome."[5]

Once you get started, you'll find this practice becomes an enjoyable habit that you look forward to completing every day.

Expectation: Increased gratitude, sense of well-being
Location in Book: Chapter 2 (Carolyn: Blessing and Gift
                      Journal)
Book Source: *Life's Companion*, Christina Baldwin

5. Gratitude Test

Take the Greater Good Science Center (UC Berkeley) quiz to
determine your degree of gratitude.

Expectation: Determine your degree of gratitude
Location in Book: Chapter 2 (Betty: The Crystal Bowl)
Website Link: https://greatergood.berkeley.edu/quizzes/
                      take_quiz/gratitude

6. Joy Buddy

Identify a special person in your life, either a family member
or a friend. This activity is more effective if that someone has
the same positive attitude towards life and aging as you do.
Get together with them often—over coffee, lunch, or online
if a face-to-face meeting is not possible—to share your
thoughts of gratitude. For example, if you do this weekly,
begin with one of you outlining the most joyful thing that
has happened to you since you last spoke. Take turns going
through your list of gratitude events and see how long you
can keep the conversation going. Just remember—no negative thoughts are allowed during these "joy chats."

Expectation: Increased gratitude, sense of well-being
Location in Book: Chapter 2 (Gratitude section)

POSITIVITY/OPTIMISM

7. 4 Ways to Increase Your Confidence from the Inside Out

Angela Loeb provides some excellent advice. In her article she discusses how to:

1. Reframe Your Self-Talk
2. Watch Language
3. Use Your Body to Speak
4. Take Action

Expectation: Increased confidence
Location in Book: Chapter 6 (Polly: From Introversion to Volunteerism)
Website Link: https://beradiantsquared.com/increase-confidence

8. Character Strengths and Virtues

The book *Character Strengths and Virtues* classifies twenty-four specific strengths under six broad virtues and is the backbone of the modern science of Positive Psychology. This science focuses on strengths rather than weaknesses. You can take a survey at the link below to determine your strengths. After you've completed the survey, a very comprehensive report is prepared for you that is helpful in determining your character strengths and how they can be applied successfully in your life.

Expectation:	Identify your character strengths
Location in Book:	Chapter 1 (Marie: The Word in Her Heart)
	Chapter 1 (Kathy: Laughing Fear in the Face)
	Chapter 2 (Betty: The Crystal Bowl Revisited)
	Chapter 5 (Wisdom section)
Book Source:	*Character Strengths and Virtues*, Christopher Peterson and Martin Seligman
Website Link:	https://www.viacharacter.org/survey/account/register

9. Explanatory Style

Martin Seligman defines *explanatory style* as the manner in which you habitually explain to yourself why events happen. He refers to a "word in your heart," a "no" or a "yes" that determines your level of pessimism or optimism. A process to determine the "word in your heart" is embedded in *Inclined Elders*.

Expectation:	Determine your level of optimism vs pessimism
Location in Book:	Chapter 1 (Marie: The Word in Her Heart)

Book Source: *Learned Optimism*, Martin Seligman and
                      Authentic Happiness, Martin Seligman

10. Law of Attraction

While there is controversy as to whether the Law of Attraction is based in science or not, I opt to believe that it is. To me it just makes sense. It aligns with the power of positive thinking that is supported by scientific studies in books such as:

- *The Law of Attraction*: Esther and Jerry Hicks
- *Authentic Happiness*: Martin Seligman
- *Learned Optimism*: Martin Seligman
- *Positivity*: Barbara Fredrickson
- *The Primer of Positive Psychology*: Christopher Peterson
- *The Secret*: Rhonda Byrne

So what is the Law of Attraction? The law is the belief that thoughts can change a person's life either positively or negatively. This concept isn't new. In his book *Think and Grow Rich* in 1937, Napoleon Hill popularized the notion and refers to our ability to attract the things we focus on into our lives.[6] The classic, *The Power of Positive Thinking* by Norman Vincent Peale, was first published in 1952. In 1956, in *The Strangest Secret,* Earl Nightingale asserted, "We become what we think about"[7] or we become our thoughts.

Personally, I find it powerful medicine, and I take it in strong doses. My current favorites are the teachings of Abraham-Hicks and Mike Dooley's Notes from the Universe—links to subscribe to both daily emails are included below.

A friend recently shared with me that one of the things she has always found helpful in shifting thoughts into things is Mike Dooley's advice to gaze from, not upon, the life you want to inhabit. By which he means, act as if you already have the life you want and go about your business accordingly. That's a much more powerful way to "trick" the brain, rather than always gazing at something you want but don't have right now.

Expectation: Increased positivity
Location in Book: Chapter 1 (Carol: The Dancer)
Website Link: Abraham-Hicks: www.abraham-hicks.com
                             Notes from the Universe: www.tut.com/
                             inspiration/nftu/

11. Mindfulness

The following "mindfulness solutions" are provided at the link below:

- Free Guided Meditations
- Mindfulness Meditation
- Meditation Audio
- Mindfulness Training
- Relaxation Techniques

Expectation: Increased overall well-being
Location in Book: Chapter 1 (Terry: Living in the Now)
Website Link: www.mindfulness-solutions.com

12. Positive Affirmations

Positive affirmations are positive statements that can help you challenge and overcome self-sabotage and negative thoughts. When you repeat them often and believe in them, you can start to make positive changes in your life. This can be a very powerful and transforming process.

IMPORTANT: Always frame the affirmations as if you already are experiencing what you are seeking.

Every day as part of my morning ritual, after my meditation, I recite to myself a litany of positive affirmations. Examples are included below.

Source: Convent Retreat
In the early 1980s, I had the good fortune to attend a weekend retreat at a local convent. The nuns held a workshop on living a meaningful and purposeful life to create inner happiness. The strongest takeaway for me was the following series of affirmations that I recite to myself every morning. While I have tweaked them slightly over the years, the overall essence remains intact. I started repeating this series in my twenties, and I'm still using it today as I head into my seventh decade. These affirmations continue to serve me well as I continue to live a life of Incline.

I love myself unconditionally and I enjoy
being the special and unique person I am.
I never devalue myself with destructive self-criticism.
I have unconditional warm regard for
all persons at all times.
I habitually speak, think, and act with
enthusiasm and positivity.
I am completely self-directed and allow
others the same right.
I take total responsibility for all my actions.

Source: The Secret
In her book *The Secret*, Rhonda Byrne maintains that the
following seven words create the strongest affirmations:

I'm so happy and grateful that I am:
Happy
Harmonious
Loving
Perfect
Powerful
Strong
Whole[8]

THEN ADD YOUR OWN PERSONAL ONES:
I'm so happy and grateful that I am:

A FEW OF MINE ARE:

I'm so happy and grateful that I experience true
freedom to be, do, and achieve all I desire as
I awaken to my spiritual nature.
I'm so happy and grateful that I live my life with
authenticity, intention, and mindfulness.
I'm so happy and grateful I'm aware that what I seek is
already in me and my power and joy are within.

CONSIDER THE FOLLOWING AS YOU BEGIN TO
EMBRACE A LIFE OF INCLINE

I'm so happy and grateful I made the choice to commit
to a meaningful, purposeful life of Incline as I get older.
I'm so happy and grateful I wake up every morning
with a plan to make each day count.
I'm so happy and grateful I live life
with a positive attitude.
I'm so happy and grateful I'm involved in
some form of movement activity every day.
I'm so happy and grateful I'm living my best life
serving as a role model for future generations.

Expectation: Increased positivity to continue to be, do,
                   achieve your desires as you age
Location in Book: Chapter 1 (Choices section)

13. Positivity Ratio

Take the Positivity Text to determine your Positivity Ratio. Further information is embedded in the book text in chapter 1.

Expectation: Increased positivity
Location in Book: Chapter 1 (Carolyn: The Dancer)
Book Source: *Positivity*, Barbara Fredrickson
Website Link: http://www.positivityratio.com/single.php

14. Self-Compassion Test

Take the test below to determine your scores in:

- Self-Kindness
- Self-Judgment
- Common Humanity
- Isolation
- Mindfulness
- Over-identification
- Overall score

Expectation: Self-compassion awareness
Location in Book: Chapter 6 (Self-Empowerment section)
Website Link: https://self-compassion.org/
                           test-how-self-compassionate-you-are/

15. Thriving Test

Take Barbara Waxman's Thriving Test to determine if:

- You are thriving
- You are nearly thriving
- You are in the 'blah' zone
- You are sputtering
- You are depleted

Expectation: Determine your degree of thriving
Location in Book: Chapter 4 (Life Course—Middlescence)
Book Source: *The Middlescence Manifesto*, Barbara
                   Waxman
Website Link: https://barbarawaxman.com/
                   thethrivingquiz/

PURPOSE

16. Ikigai

Ikigai is a Japanese practice aimed at creating life balance. It's a lifestyle that strives to balance the spiritual with the practical. The term roughly translated means "a reason for being," a sense of purpose, or "a reason for getting up in the morning." Ikigai originated on the island of Okinawa, known as one of the world's longevity hotspots where centenarians abound. In addition to eating habits and living environment, Ikigai is attributed to play a major role in aging healthily. One of the primary reasons is because it makes it possible to keep looking forward, towards the future.

The life balance is found at the intersection of four elements:

- Mission: what the world needs
- Passion: what you love
- Profession: what you are good at
- Vocation: what you can be paid for

It's proposed that having a clearly defined Ikigai can bring satisfaction, happiness, meaning, and purpose to our lives. In Japan people continue to be active after they retire. Interestingly, in Japanese there is no word that means retire.[9]

Expectation: Increased sense of purpose
Location in Book: Chapter 2 (Purpose section)
Book Source: *Ikigai*, Hector Garcia and Francesc Miralles

17. The Art of Contemplation

Richard Rudd defines the art of contemplation as a journey, an inner voyage, an adventure into the nature of your own consciousness, and the process is referred to as self-illumination. It definitely has lightened and brightened my ongoing inner path and in turn my external journey.

The ultimate goal of contemplation is to bring both our inner and outer lives into balance. Rudd further clarifies that the art of contemplation is as old as the hills and we still do it today—often unknowingly. What I found especially unique about this approach is the use of three simple progressive techniques: Pausing—related to the mind; Pivoting—related to the emotions; and Merging—related to the physical body.

Contemplation can be practiced in many ways: movement, walking, running, sitting, serving tea, or being in nature, to name a few. Since becoming more aware of the properties for increased self-awareness, I have used them with great success in several of these ways. I highly recommend exploring Richard Rudd's process in *The Art of Contemplation.*

Expectation: Increased self-illumination and sense of
                          purpose
Location in Book: Chapter 2 (Purpose section)
Book Source: *The Art of Contemplation,* Richard Rudd

CONTRIBUTORS

I would like to thank everyone who kindly agreed to be interviewed for this book and allowed me to include their stories. There are those who contributed but wish to remain anonymous for various reasons and I have respected their wishes. In addition to these anonymous individuals, I would like to thank the following people:

Amanda Jane Avis: Amanda Jane believes that movement is medicine and that we ALL have the physical intelligence to become strong and flexible at ANY age! She adores guiding her clients to where they wish to be and BEYOND! www.malamotion.com Phoenix, Arizona.

Andrea Wiggins: Andrea is a women's fitness coach who is passionate about empowering women to break up with their limiting beliefs and embrace the beauty in their strength, both in their bodies and in their lives. www.andreawigginsstrong.com Austin, Texas.

Angela Loeb: Angela enjoys working with professionals on the threshold of career decision and transition. She's also a professional speaker and writer. More at https://Insync Resources.com Lago Vista, Texas.

Betty Schroader: Betty is a survivor of two major Louisiana hurricanes and numerous surgeries. With a smile always on her face, she is grateful for all the blessings in her life. Austin, Texas.

Bill McGrath: Bill, a Parkinson's patient, is a member of the Capital Area Parkinson's Society and Power for Parkinson's. Austin, Texas.

BJ Garcia: BJ is an international best-selling author and inspirational teacher. She loves sharing with others all the many strands of interest and wisdom she has collected and moved through in her personal journey for truth. Her deep love is sharing the Gene Keys Transmission. www.bjgarcia. com Austin, Texas.

Briana Loeb: Briana resides in Austin, Texas.

Carolyn Joy Scheider: After earning her master's degree from the University of Iowa, Carolyn Joy taught in public schools from coast to coast, served as a church organist, and taught private piano lessons. In retirement, Carolyn facilitated a story circle where she wrote down her stories and encouraged others to do the same. She still has a passion for writing her life's stories. Now at eighty, she enjoys life more than ever and tries to make every day count. Austin, Texas.

Chris and Ashley Oliver: Chris and Ashley reside in Granum, Alberta, Canada.

Colin Rutner: Colin is a medical student at Texas A & M University. He starts his residency in radiology in 2020. He also is a drummer and practices yoga. Austin, Texas.

Darlene Templeton: Darlene Templeton is a dynamic professional speaker, CEO, and founder of Templeton & Associates, Amazing Women Alliance, and Amazing Women Leaders. Her business is your success and growth. These groups include high-achieving women who inspire, motivate, and support each other to achieve their goals in person and virtually through the Amazing Women Alliance Member Circle. Templeton's unique combination of extensive corporate experience (thirty-six years at IBM) and her personal career journey have given her the ability to work with professional women, individuals, businesses, and Fortune 100 companies to help define their goals, enhance performance, and achieve outstanding results. www.amazingwomenalliance.com Austin, Texas.

Darryle Clott: Darryle lives by George Bernard Shaw's words, "I am of the opinion that my life belongs to the community...and as long as I live, it is my privilege to do for it whatever I can. I want to be thoroughly used up when I die, for the harder I work, the more I live." La Crosse, Wisconsin.

David Reed: David is humbled and honored to be considered an Incliner. His faith is his guidepost and community is faith in action. Austin, Texas.

Dora Perez: Dora is a Hispanic woman who works in higher education. She was born in California to parents who were migrant labor workers. When she was four years old, her family moved to the Rio Grande Valley of south Texas, thirty miles from the Mexican border. Dora experienced an upbringing with little means, though rich in traditions, and a culture that highly valued religion, humility, family, and great respect for their elders. Austin, Texas.

Dorie Dillard: Dorie is a believer of building relationships and meaningful connections as she guides clients through the process of making important decisions in buying and selling residential real estate. It's a beautiful thing—her career and passion have come together. She loves what she does! www.canyoncreeknews.com and www.reloaustin.com Austin, Texas.

Edith Troen: Edith is a co-founder of Austin Yoga Tree and the creator of Kids Life Mastery, a program that teaches children the resiliency tools necessary to live a truly success-ful life. After spending many years in the medical industry helping sick people get healthy, she now helps others before they get sick. With a daily dose of courage, accep-tance, kindness, and self-compassion, Edith helps herself and her clients live healthy and wealthy lives every day. https://www.kidslifemastery.com Austin, Texas.

Fran and Bill Virun: Living life and looking for fun no matter their age. Currently managing their photography business, Visually Attractive Photography. www.visually attractive.com Austin, Texas.

Galen Metz: Galen is the author of *Unlock the Secrets of Retirement* and *Unlock the Secrets of Retirement Workbook*. While much has been written on financial readiness for retire-ment, these are the first books to provide an easy-to-use, step-by-step, how-to process called CARPE VITAM (Latin for "Seize Life") for planning your dream life as an Inclined Elder. Retired after thirty years of healthcare IT leader-ship, Galen now follows his retirement plan as an author, speaker, consultant, and magician. Madison, Wisconsin.

Hailey Stout: Hailey resides in New York City, New York.

Herb Stern: Herb is an Eternal Incliner and resides in Austin, Texas.

Ian Rutner: Ian is a data scientist. He also plays the hurdy gurdy and practices yoga. Austin, Texas.

Jim Opre: Jim is continually trying new and different areas of interest. He enjoys looking back at what he has accomplished and looking forward to new adventures. His interests span astronomy, woodworking, community service, and fire/rescue services. Etoile, Texas.

Jody Elrod: Jody resides in Austin, Texas.

Jonathan Troen: Jonathan is a Life Mastery Coach, co-founder of Austin Yoga Tree and creator of Self Love Revolution. He spent twenty-five years in the entertainment industry, searching for the admiration of others, before discovering all he really needed to master true success was to love himself. His new mission in life: to help people find the joy inside of themselves. Learn more at www.Troen.net or www.SelfLoveRevolution.com Austin, Texas.

Judy Kuipers: Dr. Kuipers' career culminated in twenty years as president of two universities where she sought to advance the contributions that higher education makes to individual lives, communities, and to the world. Fresno, California.

Julie Wylie: Julie uses her eclectic background in Somatic Movement Practices including Nia Technique and tai chi to create comfortable, safe spaces for individuals to find health, healing, and well-being. She contributes to the greater good as a volunteer facilitator of movement, creative writing, and public speaking classes in women's prisons around Central Texas. www.JulieAnnWylie.com Austin, Texas.

Kathy Mohler: A nurse, wife, mother, and friend. Always passionate about advocacy for the aging population and maintaining a zest for life. Her motto is "I'm never going to grow up." Austin, Texas.

Kristin Huber: Kristin is a mid-to-late career professional seeking to learn from her active mentors and family members as role models to build the right skills and mindset to launch her "next act." Austin, Texas.

Lee Moczygemba: At fifty Lee began a successful career as an inspiring international motivational speaker and is now the oldest living member of the National Speakers Association. In 2013 she was awarded the Lifetime Achievement Award by the National Speakers Association Austin Chapter. Her inner child is alive and kicking in her ninety-fifth year. Austin, Texas.

Nancy Jones: Nancy says: "You're as young as you feel." She is in her third career and loving life! Austin, Texas.

Nancy Stern Bain: Nancy is a dance educator, choreographer, and dancer. Currently, she teaches dance to people with Parkinson's Disease. Austin, Texas.

Phyllis Books: Dr. Books definitely tries not to "act her age" and surprises most everyone with her eagerness level and her curiosity. She is always up for a new adventure and new research to back up her theories and trademarked techniques using neuroscience advances. She lectures and trains people how to activate new potentials and learning possibilities in children of any age. www.drphyllisbooks. com Austin, Texas.

Polly Enders: Polly resides in Austin, Texas.

Raymond Oliver: Always "feet forward," an Army Reserve term meaning eagerness, ambition, determination, and a positive outlook. Vernon, British Columbia, Canada.

Steve and Bobbi-Jo Oliver: Steve and Bobbi-Jo reside in Vernon, British Columbia, Canada.

Suzanne Oliver: A proud sister to a "super sister," Ramona. We're Inclining together. Vernon, British Columbia, Canada.

Terry Morganti Fisher: Harnessing a lifetime of experience as an elder, educator, and body-centered coach, Terry catalyzes opportunities for women to inspire multigenerational transformation for the common good. www.women growingbolder.com Austin, Texas.

Tracy Williams: Opposed to the term retirement, Tracy is redirected from her thirty-three-year career in education and has embarked on a new career in the arts, including sculpture and Ikebana floral arranging. An avid traveller, she looks forward to new adventures and believes in a progressive approach to aging. Instagram: @awesometracy 1127. Austin, Texas.

WellMed Senior Center: a senior community center in Austin, Texas.

- Valerie Castillo resides in Austin, Texas.
- John Pratt resides in Austin, Texas.
- Jimmy Isaacson resides in Austin, Texas.
- Gregory Cantu resides in Austin, Texas.
- Uwe Ehlers resides in Austin, Texas.

.

ABOUT THE AUTHOR

Ramona Oliver has long been passionate about supporting individuals with their personal and professional development. As a septuagenarian, this passion is now directed toward positive aging.

Formerly, Ramona has taken on roles including human resource manager/director, career coach, and director of outreach. As a human resource director for many years, she championed the professional development of employees. While serving as president of the Austin Human Resource Management Association, she led an award-winning team that designed, developed, and implemented a leadership program. In addition, she launched a workforce readiness committee that partnered with community organizations to implement workforce readiness initiatives. At St. Edward's University, she promoted the adult undergraduate and graduate programs to older adults in the Austin community.

Ramona currently serves as an advocate of positive aging. Rather than accepting a mindset of decline, Ramona is passionate about living life with an attitude of Incline.

She has been published on the Changing Aging website, offering posts with titles such as "Can We Please Stop Calling It Aging," "What Are We Missing When We Settle for Life Stages?" and "Leave a Legacy and Live It Now!" She earned her Master of Business Administration from St. Edward's University.

Ramona lives in Austin, Texas. Her website is www.ramonavmoliver.com.

NOTES

Introduction

1 "Life expectancy in North America 2019," Statista, accessed February 28, 2020, https://www.statista.com/statistics/274513/life-expectancy-in-north-america/.

2 Isla Rippon and Andrew Steptoe, "Feeling Old vs being Old: Associations Between Self-Perceived Age and Mortality," *JAMA Network* (February 2015): https://jamanetwork.com/journals/jamainternalmedicine/fullarticle/2020288.

Chapter One

1 Ellen Langer, *Counterclockwise* (New York, NY: Ballantine Books, 2009), chap. 1, Kindle.

2 Martin Seligman, *Learned Optimism* (New York, NY: Vintage Books, 2006), chap. 1, Kindle.

3 Seligman, *Learned Optimism,* chap. 1.

4 Christopher Peterson and Martin Seligman, *Character Strengths and Virtues* (New York, NY: Oxford University Press, 2004), chap. 1, Kindle.

5 Martin Seligman, *Learned Optimism* (New York, NY: Vintage Books, 2006), chap. 3, Kindle.

6 Barbara Fredrickson, *Positivity* (New York, NY: Three Rivers Press, 2009), chap. 2, Kindle.

7 Esther and Jerry Hicks, *The Law of Attraction* (Carlsbad, CA: Hay House, 2006), Part II, Kindle.

8 Kathrin Rehfeld, "Dancing or Fitness Sport?" *Frontiers in Human Neuroscience* (June 2017): https://www.frontiersin.org/articles/10.3389/fnhum.2017.00305/full.

9 Gene D. Cohen, *The Mature Mind* (New York, NY: Basic Books, 2005), chap. 1, Kindle.

10 Cohen, *The Mature Mind,* chap. 1.

11 Norman Doidge, *The Brain That Changes Itself* (New York, NY: Penguin Books, 2007), Preface, Kindle.

12 Florence Williams, *The 3-Day Effect* (Audible Original: Audible, 2018)

13 Florence Williams, "This is Your Brain on Nature," *National Geographic* (January 2016): https://www.nationalgeographic.com/magazine/2016/01/call-to-wild/.

14 Qing Li, *Forest Bathing* (New York, NY: Viking, 2018), Introduction, Kindle.

15 Ellen Langer, *Counterclockwise* (New York, NY: Ballantine Books, 2009), chap. 1, Kindle.

16 George Loewenstein, "The Psychology of Curiosity: A Review and Reinterpretation," *Psychological Bulletin* Vol 116. No. 1 (1994): https://pdfs.semanticscholar.org/f946/7adac17f3ef6d65cdcf38b46afb974abfa55.pdf.

17 Erik Wahl, *Unthink: Rediscover Your Creative Genius* (New York, NY: Crown Business, 2013), Introduction, Kindle.

18 William Clark, "Is our tendency to experience fear and anxiety genetic?" Scientific American, March 6, 2000, https://www.scientificamerican.com/article/is-our-tendency-to-experi/.

19 Brené Brown, *Daring Greatly* (New York, NY: Avery, 2012), chap. 4, Kindle.

20 Dave Cornell, "3 Lessons on Courage from The Wizard of Oz," Cultivate Courage, September 30, 2019, http://www.cultivatecourage.com/3-lessons-on-courage-from-the-wizard-of-oz/.

Chapter Two

1 Madhuleena Roy Chowdhury, "The Neuroscience of Gratitude and How It Affects Anxiety & Grief," PositivePsychology.com, September 4, 2019, https://positivepsychology.com/neuroscience-of-gratitude/.

2 "Gratitude Quiz," Greater Good Science Center at UC Berkeley, accessed March 2, 2020, https://greatergood.berkeley.edu/quizzes/take_quiz/gratitude.

3 Angela Loeb, "3 Good Things," *Insync Resources* (blog), June 7, 2018, https://www.linkedin.com/pulse/3-good-things-angela-loeb.

4 Christina Baldwin, *Life's Companion* (New York, NY: Bantam Dell, 1991), 180.

5 Martin Seligman, *Authentic Happiness* (New York, NY: Free Press, 2002), Preface, Kindle.

6 Christopher Peterson and Martin Seligman, *Character Strengths and Virtues* (New York, NY: Oxford University Press, 2004), chap. 3, Kindle.

7 Sue Treiman and Amit Sood, MD, "Q&A About Finding Resilience to Chronic Stress Through Neuroscience," Everyday Health, February 14, 2019, https://www.everydayhealth.com/wellness/united-states-of-stress/advisory-board/amit-sood-md-q-a/.

8 Barbara Fredrickson, *Positivity* (New York, NY: Three Rivers Press, 2008), chap. 6, Kindle.

9 Robert Glazer, "Resilience and Gratitude," *Friday Forward* (blog), October 7, 2016, https://www.robertglazer.com/friday-forward/resilience-control-gratitude/.

10 Richard Rudd, *Gene Keys* (London, England, Watkins Publishing, 2013), Kindle.

11 Rudd, *Gene Keys*.

12 Richard Rudd, *The Art of Contemplation* (Poole, UK: Gene Keys Publishing Ltd., 2018).

13 Victor Frankl, *Man's Search for Meaning* (Boston, MA: Beacon Press, 2006), chap. 1, Kindle.

14 Aliya Alimujiang, "Association Between Life Purpose and Mortality Among US Adults Older Than 50 Years," *JAMA Network Open* (May 24, 2019): https://jamanetwork.com/journals/jamanetworkopen/fullarticle/2734064.

15 "Purpose in the Encore Years," *Encore.org*, Accessed April 20, 2018, p. 5, https://encore.org/wp-content/uploads/2018/03/PEP-Full-Report.pdf.

16 "Amazing Women Alliance," accessed February 23, 2020, https://amazingwomenalliance.com/.

Chapter Three

1 Stuart Brown with Christopher Vaughan, *Play* (New York, NY: Penguin Group, 2009), chap. 1, Kindle.

2 Stuart and Vaughan, *Play,* chap. 2.

3 Stuart and Vaughan, *Play,* chap. 2.

4 Stuart and Vaughan, *Play,* chap. 3.

5 Tanner Christensen, "Why Play is Essential for Creativity," CreativeSomething.net, April 28, 2014, https://creativesomething.net/post/84134598535/why-play-is-essential-for-creativity.

6 Stuart Brown with Christopher Vaughan, *Play* (New York, NY: Penguin Group, 2009), chap. 2, Kindle.

7 Stuart and Vaughan, *Play,* chap. 2.

8 "Amanda Jane Avis is Malamotion," Malamotion, accessed February 29, 2020, http://www.malamotion.com/.

9 Simon Gandevia and Uwe Proske, "Proprioception: The Sense Within," *The Scientist* (August 31, 2016): https://www.the-scientist.com/features/proprioception-the-sense-within-32940.

10 "Physical Activity Program Helps Maintain Mobility," National Institute of Health, June 2, 2014, https://www.nih.gov/news-events/nih-research-matters/physical-activity-program-helps-maintain-mobility.

11 Mihaly Csikszentmihalyi, *Flow and the Foundations of Positive Psychology* (Dordrecht, Netherlands: Springer, 2014), chap. 1, Kindle.

12 Csikszentmihalyi, *Flow and the Foundations of Positive Psychology,* Preface.

13 Csikszentmihalyi, *Flow and the Foundations of Positive Psychology*, chap. 9.

14 Debbie and Carlos Rosas, *The Nia Technique* (New York, NY: Broadway Books, 2004), 17.

15 Kathrin Rehfeld, "Dancing or Fitness Sport?" *Frontiers in Human Neuroscience* (June 2017): https://www.frontiersin.org/articles/10.3389/fnhum.2017.00305/full.

16 "About Us," Power for Parkinson's, accessed February 29, 2020, https://www.powerfor parkinsons.org/about-us.

17 Julia Cameron, *It's Never Too Late to Begin Again,* (New York, NY: TarcherPerigee, 2016), Cover.

18 Gene Cohen, *The Creative Age* (New York, NY: Avon Books, 2000), 11.

19 "Mission," National Center for Creative Aging, accessed February 29, 2020, https://creativeaging.org.

20 Rohini Venkatraman, "Science Says We Get Less Creative as We Age. Prove It Wrong by Doing 1 of These 3 Things," Inc.com, August 29, 2017, https://www.inc.com/rohini-venkatraman/science-says-we-get-less-creative-as-we-age-prove-.html.

21 Gene Cohen, "Research on Creativity and Aging," *Generations* 30 (1) (Spring 2006): accessed March 6, 2020, https://www.agingkingcounty.org/wp-content/uploads/sites/185/2016/07/RESEARCH-ON-CREATIVITY-AND-AGING.pdf.

22 Cohen, "Research on Creativity and Aging."

23 Cohen, "Research on Creativity and Aging."

24 Gene Cohen, "The Creativity and Aging Study," National Endowment for the Arts, April 30, 2006, https://www.arts.gov/sites/default/files/NEA-Creativity-and-Aging-Cohen-study.pdf.

Chapter Four

1 "Aging Well, The Harvard Study," Namaste Connections, March 10, 2018, https://www.namasteconnections.com/single-post/2018/03/10/Aging-Well-The-Harvard-Study.

2 "Aging Well, The Harvard Study," Namaste Connections.

3 "Aging Well, The Harvard Study," Namaste Connections.

4 "#Other People Matter," The Positivity Project, accessed March 1, 2020, https://posproject.org/other-people-matter-mindset/.

5 "#Other People Matter," The Positivity Project.

6 "Social Engagement," Stanford Center on Longevity, Sight-lines Project Special Report, accessed March 1, 2020, http://longevity.stanford.edu/sightlines-project-social-engagement-special-report/.

7 Lynda Gratton and Andrew Scott, *The 100-Year Life* (London, UK: Bloomsbury, 2016), Introduction, Kindle.

8 "Life Course Theory," Encyclopedia.com, accessed March 1, 2020, https://www.encyclopedia.com/reference/encyclopedias-almanacs-transcripts-and-maps/life-course-theory.

9 Glen Elder, Jr. and Janet Giele, *The Craft of Life Course Research* (New York, NY: Guildford Publications, 2009), 11, https://www.guilford.com/excerpts/elder.pdf.

10 Caitrin Lynch and Jason Danely, ed., *Transitions and Transformations* (New York, NY: Berghahn Books, 2013), Introduction, Kindle.

11 Amy Wilkinson, "The Surprising (Relative Old) Age of Entrepreneurs," *The Wall Street Journal*, January 29,

2015, https://blogs.wsj.com/experts/2015/01/29/the-surprising-relatively-old-age-of-entrepreneurs/.

12 Barbara Waxman, *The Middlescence Manifesto* (Kentfield, CA: The Middlescence Factor, 2016), chap. 5, Kindle.

13 Waxman, *The Middlescence Manifesto,* chap. 5.

14 Elizabeth D. Hutchison, *Dimensions of Human Behavior* (Thousand Oaks, CA: Sage Publications, Inc., 2019), Kindle.

15 Hutchison, *Dimensions of Human Behavior.*

16 Elizabeth Harvey, "What's Generativity and Why It's Good for You," Huffington Post, June 23, 2016, https://www.huffpost.com/entry/whats-generativity-and-why-its-good-for-you_b_7629174.

17 Stephanie Firestone, "Incentivizing Multigenerational Living," *Thinking Policy* (blog), AARP, May 23, 2019, https://blog.aarp.org/thinking-policy/incentivizing-multigenerational-living.

18 Stephanie Firestone, "Incentivizing Multigenerational Living."

19 Stephanie Firestone, "Incentivizing Multigenerational Living."

20 "Our Core Values," Encore.org, accessed February 29, 2020, https://encore.org/our-team/.

21 Marc Freeman, *How to Live Forever* (New York, NY: Public Affairs Books, 2018), Introduction, Kindle.

Chapter Five

1 John Monaghan and Peter Just, *Social and Cultural Anthropology* (New York, NY: Oxford University Press, 2000), chap. 2, Kindle.

2 Managhan and Just, *Social and Cultural Anthropology,* chap. 2.

3 "Differences Between Culture and Society," KPU Differences, August 12, 2017, https://keydifferences.com/difference-between-culture-and-society.html.

4 Jay Sokolovsky, ed., *The Cultural Context of Aging* (Westport, CT: Praeger Publishers, 2009), Introduction, Kindle.

5 Uri Friedman, "The End of the Age Pyramid," *The Atlantic,* June 28, 2014, https://www.theatlantic.com/international/archive/2014/06/the-shifting-shape-of-age-around-the-world/373638/.

6 Caitrin Lynch and Jason Danely, ed., *Transitions and Transformations* (New York, NY: Berghahn Books, 2013), chap. 11, Kindle.

7 Lynch and Danely, *Transitions and Transformations,* chap. 11.

8 Lynch and Danely, *Transitions and Transformations,* chap. 11.

9 Nidhi Sharma, "Daughter-in-law & Son-in-law too would be responsible for care of old," *The Economic Times*, April 14, 2018, https://economictimes.indiatimes.com/news/politics-and-nation/daughter-in-law-son-in-law-too-would-be-responsible-for-care-of-old/articleshow/63756469.cms

10 Heizo Takenaka, "Elderly workers: Expectations and challenges," *The Japan Times*, March 26, 2019, https://www.japantimes.co.jp/opinion/2019/03/26/commentary/japan-commentary/elderly-workers-expectations-challenges/.

11 Isabel Reynolds and Emi Nobuhiro, "Job seekers in their 70s could become Japan's new normal," *The Japan Times,* May 23, 2019, https://www.japantimes.co.jp/news/2019/05/23/national/social-issues/septuagenarian-job-hunters-become-japans-new-normal/.

12 Colin Joyce, "Japan moves to protect the elderly," *Telegraph,* November 2, 2005, https://www.telegraph.co.uk/news/worldnews/asia/japan/1502071/Japan-moves-to-protect-the-elderly.html.

13 Ruth Walker, "Elder Abuse Legislation," *Missouri State Gerontology Program,* January 13, 2019, https://blogs.missouristate.edu/gerontology/2019/01/13/elder-abuse-legislation-japan-vs-the-united-states/.

14 Dan Buettner, *The Blue Zones, Second Edition* (Washington, D.C.: National Geographic Society, 2012), Reflecting on the Lessons, Conclusion, Kindle.

15 "Grumpy Old Men No More," Stanford Center on Longevity, November 12, 2007, http://longevity.stanford.edu/2011/06/21/111207-grumpy-old-men-no-more/.

16 Lucy Rock, "Life Gets Better after 50: why age tends to work in favour of happiness," *The Guardian,* May 5, 2018, https://www.theguardian.com/lifeandstyle/2018/may/05/happiness-curve-life-gets-better-after-50-jonathan-rauch.

17 "Debunking the Double Standard on Aging in Men vs. Women," *Joylux,* accessed March 8, 2020, https://joylux.com/blogs/news/debunking-the-double-standard-on-aging-in-men-vs-women.

18 Christopher Peterson and Martin Seligman, *Character Strengths and Virtues* (New York, NY: Oxford University Press, 2004), chap. 4, Kindle.

19 Peterson and Seligman, *Character Strengths and Virtues,* chap. 4.

20 Ryan Niemiec, *Character Strength Interventions* (Boston, MA: Hogrefe Publishing, 2018), chap. 1, Kindle.

21 Adrian Farrell, "Monika Ardelt on How to Become Wise," CanDoWisdom.com, January 21, 2017, https://candowisdom. com/wisdom/monika-ardelt-become-wise.

22 Adrian Farrell, "Monika Ardelt on How to Become Wise."

Chapter Six

1 Nanette Page and Cheryl Czuba, "Empowerment: What Is It?," *The Journal of Extension* 37(5) (October 1999), https:// www.joe.org/joe/1999october/comm1.php/php.

2 Steve Bruce, *Sociology: A Very Short Introduction* (Oxford, UK, Oxford University Press, 2018), Kindle.

3 Richard Sharf, *Theories of Psychotherapy and Counseling, 5th ed.* (Belmont, CA: Brooks/Cole, 2012), 91.

4 "Extraversion and Introversion," Psychologist World, accessed March 1, 2020, https://www.psychologistworld. com/influence-personality/extraversion-introversion.

5 Carol Bainbridge, "The Difference Between Being Shy and Being Introverted," Very Well Family, September 15, 2019, https://www.verywellfamily.com/the-difference-between-being-shy-and-being-introverted-1448616?print.

6 Angela Loeb, "4 Ways to Increase Your Confidence from the Inside Out," *InSyncResources* (blog), accessed March 7, 2020, https://beradiantsquared.com/increase-confidence/.

7 Sharon D'Agostino, "Love and Empowerment," Say It Forward.org, February 12, 2019, https://sayitforward.org/ love-and-empowerment/.

8 Richard Rudd, *Gene Keys* (London, UK: Watkins Publishing: 2013), Kindle.

9 Kristin Neff, "What Self-Compassion Is," Self-Compassion.com, accessed March 7, 2020, https://self-compassion.org/the-three-elements-of-self-compassion-2/.

10 Neff, "What Self-Compassion Is."

11 Paul Irving, "Self-Empowerment in Later Life as a Response to Ageism," American Society on Aging, accessed March 1, 2020, https://www.asaging.org/blog/self-empowerment-later-life-response-ageism.

12 Stephanie Firestone, "Incentivizing Multigenerational Living," *Thinking Policy* (blog), AARP, May 23, 2019, https://blog.aarp.org/thinking-policy/incentivizing-multigenerational-living.

13 Firestone, "Incentivizing Multigenerational Living."

14 "That Age Old Question," Royal Society for Public Health, accessed March 7, 2020, https://www.rsph.org.uk/our-work/policy/older-people/that-age-old-question.html.

15 Jacob Banas, "Disrupting the Reaper," Futurism, October 12, 2018, https://futurism.com/live-forever-silicon-valley.

16 Ezekiel Emanuel, "Why I Hope to Die at 75," *The Atlantic,* October 2014, https://www.theatlantic.com/magazine/archive/2014/10/why-i-hope-to-die-at-75/379329/.

17 Lynda Gratton and Andrew Scott, *The 100-Year Life,* (London, UK: Bloomsbury, 2016, Introduction, Kindle.

18 DK Digital Publishing Team, *The Sociology Book,* (New York, NY: DK Publishing, 2015), Introduction, Kindle.

19 "A New Map of Life," Stanford Center on Longevity, accessed March 1, 2020, http://longevity.stanford.edu/a-new-map-of-life.

20 "A New Map of Life," Stanford Center on Longevity.

21 "A New Map of Life," Stanford Center on Longevity.

22 "A New Map of Life," Stanford Center on Longevity.

Resources

1 Julia Cameron, *It's Never Too Late to Begin Again* (New York, NY: A TarcherPerigee Book, 2016), xviii.

2 Julia Cameron, *It's Never Too Late to Begin Again,* xix.

3 Julia Cameron, *It's Never Too Late to Begin Again,* back cover.

4 Christina Baldwin, *Life's Companion* (New York, NY: Bantam Dell, 1990), 96.

5 Christina Baldwin, *Life's Companion,* 180.

6 Napoleon Hill, *Think and Grow Rich* (Anderson, SC: The Mindpower Press, 2015), Kindle.

7 Earl Nightingale, *The Strangest Secret* (Melrose, FL: Laurenzana Press, 2011), Kindle.

8 Rhonda Byrne, *The Secret* (New York, NY: Atria Books, 2008), Kindle.

9 Hector Garcia and Francesc Miralles, *Ikigai* (New York, NY: Penguin Books, 2016), chap. 1, Kindle.

BIBLIOGRAPHY

"A New Map of Life." Stanford Center on Longevity, accessed March 1, 2020. http://longevity.stanford.edu/ a-new-map-of-life.

"About Us." Power for Parkinson's, accessed February 29, 2020. https://www.powerfor parkinsons.org/about-us.

"Aging Well, The Harvard Study." Namaste Connections. March 10, 2018. https://www.namasteconnections.com/ single-post/2018/03/10/Aging-Well-The-Harvard-Study.

Alimujiang, Aliya. "Association Between Life Purpose and Mortality Among US Adults Older Than 50 Years." *JAMA Network Open* (May 24, 2019). https://jamanetwork.com/journals/ jamanetworkopen/fullarticle/2734064.

"Amanda Jane Avis is Malamotion." Malamotion, accessed February 29, 2020. http://www.malamotion.com/.

"Amazing Women Alliance," accessed February 23, 2020. https://amazingwomenalliance.com/.

Bainbridge, Carol. "The Difference Between Being Shy and Being Introverted." Very Well Family. September 15, 2019. https://www.verywellfamily.com/the-difference-between-being-shy-and-being-introverted-1448616?print.

Baldwin, Christina. *Life's Companion.* New York, NY: Bantam Dell, 1991.

Banas, Jacob. "Disrupting the Reaper." Futurism. October 12, 2018. https://futurism.com/live-forever-silicon-valley.

Brown, Brené. *Daring Greatly.* New York, NY: Avery, 2012.

Brown, Stuart, with Christopher Vaughn. *Play.* New York, NY: Penguin Group, 2009.

Bruce, Steve. *Sociology: A Very Short Introduction.* Oxford, UK, Oxford University Press, 2018.

Buettner, Dan. *The Blue Zones, Second Edition.* Washington, D.C.: National Geographic Society, 2012.

Chowdhury, Madhuleena Roy. "The Neuroscience of Gratitude and How It Affects Anxiety & Grief." PositivePsychology. com. September 4, 2019. https://positivepsychology.com/neuroscience-of-gratitude/

Christensen, Tanner. "Why Play is Essential for Creativity." CreativeSomething.net. April 28, 2014. https://creativesomething. net/post/84134598535/why-play-is-essential-for-creativity.

Clark, William. "Is our tendency to experience fear and anxiety genetic?" Scientific American, March 6, 2000. https://www. scientificamerican.com/article/is-our-tendency-to-experi/.

Cohen, Gene. "Research on Creativity and Aging." *Generations* 30 (1) (Spring 2006), accessed March 6, 2020. https://www. agingkingcounty.org/wp-content/uploads/sites/185/2016/07/RESEARCH-ON-CREATIVITY-AND-AGING.pdf.

Cohen, Gene. *The Creative Age.* New York, NY: Avon Books, 2000.

Cohen, Gene. "The Creativity and Aging Study." National Endowment for the Arts. April 30, 2006. https://www.arts. gov/sites/default/files/NEA-Creativity-and-Aging-Cohen-study.pdf

Cohen, Gene. *The Mature Mind.* New York, NY: Basic Books, 2005.

Cornell, Dave. "3 Lessons on Courage from The Wizard of Oz." Cultivate Courage. September 30, 2019. http://www. cultivatecourage.com/3-lessons-on-courage-from-the-wizard-of-oz/.

Csikszentmihalyi, Mihaly. *Flow and the Foundations of Positive Psychology.* Dordrecht, Netherlands: Springer, 2014.

D'Agostino, Sharon. "Love and Empowerment." Say It Forward.org. February 12, 2019. https://sayitforward.org/ love-and-empowerment/.

"Debunking the Double Standard on Aging in Men vs. Women." *Joylux*, accessed March 8, 2020. https://joylux.com/blogs/news/ debunking-the-double-standard-on-aging-in-men-vs-women.

"Differences Between Culture and Society." KPU Differences. August 12, 2017. https://keydifferences.com/difference-between-culture-and-society.html.

DK Digital Publishing Team. *The Sociology Book.* New York, NY: DK Publishing, 2015.

Doidge, Norman. *The Brain That Changes Itself.* New York, NY: Penguin Books, 2007.

Elder, Glen, Jr. and Janet Giele. *The Craft of Life Course Research.* New York, NY: Guildford Publications, 2009. https://www. guilford.com/excerpts/elder.pdf.

Emanuel, Ezekiel. "Why I Hope to Die at 75." *The Atlantic.* October 2014. https://www.theatlantic.com/magazine/ archive/2014/10/why-i-hope-to-die-at-75/379329/.

"Extraversion and Introversion." Psychologist World. accessed March 1, 2020. https://www.psychologistworld.com/ influence-personality/extraversion-introversion.

Farrell, Adrian. "Monika Ardelt on How to Become Wise." CanDoWisdom.com, January 21, 2017. https://candowisdom. com/wisdom/monika-ardelt-become-wise.

Firestone, Stephanie. "Incentivizing Multigenerational Living." *Thinking Policy* (blog). AARP, May 23, 2019. https://blog.aarp. org/thinking-policy/incentivizing-multigenerational-living.

Frankl, Victor. *Man's Search for Meaning.* Boston, MA: Beacon Press, 2006.

Fredrickson, Barbara. *Positivity.* New York, NY: Three Rivers Press, 2009.

Freeman, Marc. *How to Live Forever.* New York, NY: Public Affairs Books, 2018.

Friedman, Uri. "The End of the Age Pyramid." *The Atlantic.* June 28, 2014. https://www.theatlantic.com/international/archive/ 2014/06/the-shifting-shape-of-age-around-the-world/373638/.

Gandevia, Simon, and Uwe Proske. "Proprioception: The Sense Within." *The Scientist* (August 31, 2016). https://www.the-scientist.com/features/proprioception-the-sense-within-32940.

Glazer, Robert. "Resilience and Gratitude." *Friday Forward* (blog), October 7, 2016. https://www.robertglazer.com/ friday-forward/resilience-control-gratitude/.

Gratton, Lynda and Andrew Scott. *The 100-Year Life.* London, UK: Bloomsbury, 2016.

"Grumpy Old Men No More." Stanford Center on Longevity. November 12, 2007. http://longevity.stanford.edu/2011/06/21/111207-grumpy-old-men-no-more/.

Harvey, Elizabeth. "What's Generativity and Why It's Good for You." Huffington Post. June 23, 2016. https://www.huffpost.com/entry/whats-generativity-and-why-its-good-for-you_b_7629174.

Hutchison, Elizabeth. *Dimensions of Human Behavior.* Thousand Oaks, CA: Sage Publications, Inc., 2019.

Irving, Paul. "Self-Empowerment in Later Life as a Response to Ageism." American Society on Aging, accessed March 1, 2020. https://www.asaging.org/blog/self-empowerment-later-life-response-ageism.

Joyce, Colin. "Japan moves to protect the elderly." *Telegraph.* November 2, 2005. https://www.telegraph.co.uk/news/worldnews/asia/japan/1502071/Japan-moves-to-protect-the-elderly.html.

Langer, Ellen. *Counterclockwise.* New York, NY: Ballantine Books, 2009.

Li, Qing. *Forest Bathing.* New York, NY: Viking, 2018.

"Life Course Theory." Encyclopedia.com, accessed March 1, 2020. https://www.encyclopedia.com/reference/encyclopedias-almanacs-transcripts-and-maps/life-course-theory.

"Life expectancy in North America 2019." Statista, accessed February 28, 2020. https://www.statista.com/statistics/274513/life-expectancy-in-north-america/.

Loeb, Angela. "3 Good Things." *Insync Resources* (blog), June 7, 2018. https://www.linkedin.com/pulse/3-good-things-angela-loeb.

Loeb, Angela. "4 Ways to Increase Your Confidence from the Inside Out." *InSyncResources* (blog), accessed March 7, 2020. https://beradiantsquared.com/increase-confidence/.

Loewenstein, George. "The Psychology of Curiosity: A Review and Reinterpretation." *Psychological Bulletin* Vol 116. No. 1 (1994). https://pdfs.semanticscholar.org/f946/7adac17f3ef6d65cdcf38b46afb974abfa55.pdf.

Lynch, Caitrin, and Jason Danely, ed. *Transitions and Transformations*. New York, NY: Berghahn Books, 2013.

"Mission." National Center for Creative Aging, accessed February 29, 2020. https://creativeaging.org.

Monaghan, John, and Peter Just. *Social and Cultural Anthropology*. New York, NY: Oxford University Press, 2000.

Neff, Kristin. "What Self-Compassion Is." Self-Compassion.com, accessed March 7, 2020. https://self-compassion.org/the-three-elements-of-self-compassion-2/.

Niemiec, Ryan. *Character Strength Interventions*. Boston, MA: Hogrefe Publishing, 2018.

"#Other People Matter." The Positivity Project, accessed March 1, 2020. https://posproject.org/other-people-matter-mindset/.

"Our Core Values." Encore.org, accessed February 29, 2020. https://encore.org/our-team/.

Page, Nanette, and Cheryl Czuba. "Empowerment: What Is It?" *The Journal of Extension* 37(5) (October 1999). https://www.joe.org/joe/1999october/comm1.php/php

Peterson, Christopher, and Martin Seligman. *Character Strengths and Virtues.* New York, NY: Oxford University Press, 2004.

"Physical Activity Program Helps Maintain Mobility." National Institute of Health. June 2, 2014. https://www.nih.gov/news-events/nih-research-matters/physical-activity-program-helps-maintain-mobility.

"Purpose in the Encore Years." *Encore.org,* accessed April 20, 2018, p. 5. https://encore.org/wp-content/uploads/2018/03/PEP-Full-Report.pdf.

Rehfeld, Kathrin. "Dancing or Fitness Sport?" *Frontiers in Human Neuroscience,* June 2017. https://www.frontiersin.org/articles/10.3389/fnhum.2017.00305/full.

Reynolds, Isabel, and Emi Nobuhiro. "Job seekers in their 70s could become Japan's new normal," *The Japan Times,* May 23, 2019. https://www.japantimes.co.jp/news/2019/05/23/national/social-issues/septuagenarian-job-hunters-become-japans-new-normal/.

Rippon, Isla, and Andrew Steptoe. "Feeling Old vs being Old: Associations Between Self-Perceived Age and Mortality." *JAMA Network* (February 2015). https://jamanetwork.com/journals/jamainternalmedicine/fullarticle/2020288.

Rock, Lucy. "Life gets better after 50." *The Guardian.* May 5, 2018. https://www.theguardian.com/lifeandstyle/2018/may/05/happiness-curve-life-gets-better-after-50-jonathan-rauch.

Rosas, Debbie, and Carlos Rosas. *The Nia Technique.* New York, NY: Broadway Books, 2004.

Rudd, Richard. *Gene Keys.* London, England, Watkins Publishing, 2013.

Seligman, Martin. *Authentic Happiness.* New York, NY: Free Press, 2002.

Seligman, Martin. *Learned Optimism.* New York, NY: Vintage Books, 2006.

Sharf, Richard. *Theories of Psychotherapy and Counseling, 5ᵗʰ ed.* Belmont, CA: Brooks/Cole, 2012.

Sharma, Nidhi. "Daughter-in-law & Son-in-law too would be responsible for care of old." *The Economic Times.* April 14, 2018. https://economictimes.indiatimes.com/news/politics-and-nation/daughter-in-law-son-in-law-too-would-be-responsible-for-care-of-old/articleshow/63756469.cms.

"Social Engagement." Stanford Center on Longevity, Sightlines Project Special Report, accessed March 1, 2020. http://longevity.stanford.edu/sightlines-project-social-engagement-special-report/.

Sokolovsky, Jay, ed. *The Cultural Context of Aging.* Westport, CT: Praeger Publishers, 2009.

Takenaka, Heizo. "Elderly workers: Expectations and challenges." *The Japan Times.* March 26, 2019. https://www.japantimes.co.jp/opinion/2019/03/26/commentary/japan-commentary/elderly-workers-expectations-challenges/.

"That Age Old Question." Royal Society for Public Health, accessed March 7, 2020. https://www.rsph.org.uk/our-work/policy/older-people/that-age-old-question.html.

Treiman, Sue, and Amit Sood, MD. "Q&A About Finding Resilience to Chronic Stress Through Neuroscience." Everyday Health. February 14, 2019. https://www.everydayhealth.com/wellness/united-states-of-stress/advisory-board/amit-sood-md-q-a/.

Venkatraman, Robin. "Science Says We Get Less Creative as We Age. Prove It Wrong by Doing 1 of These 3 Things." Inc.com. August 29, 2017. https://www.inc.com/rohini-venkatraman/science-says-we-get-less-creative-as-we-age-prove-.html.

Wahl, Eric. *Unthink: Rediscover Your Creative Genius.* New York, NY: Crown Business, 2013.

Walker, Ruth. "Elder Abuse Legislation." Missouri State Gerontology Program. January 13, 2019. https://blogs.missouristate.edu/gerontology/2019/01/13/elder-abuse-legislation-japan-vs-the-united-states/.

Waxman, Barbara. *The Middlescence Manifesto.* Kentfield, CA: The Middlescence Factor, 2016.

Williams, Florence. *The 3-Day Effect.* Audible Original: Audible, 2018.

Wilkinson, Amy. "The Surprising (Relative Old) Age of Entrepreneurs." *The Wall Street Journal.* January 29, 2015. https://blogs.wsj.com/experts/2015/01/29/the-surprising-relatively-old-age-of-entrepreneurs/.

Williams, Florence. "This is Your Brain on Nature." National Geographic. January 2016. https://www.nationalgeographic.com/magazine/2016/01/call-to-wild/.